Workouts for Seniors

A Beginner's Guide to a Home Strength Training

Volume 1

Harry Sloan

advice. The content within this book has been derived from various sources. Please consult a licensed professional before attempting any techniques outlined in this book.

By reading this document, the reader agrees that under no circumstances is the author responsible for any losses, direct or indirect, that are incurred as a result of the use of the information contained within this document, including, but not limited to, errors, omissions, or inaccuracies.

Table of Contents

CHAPTER 5: THE TANGIBLE BENEFITS OF UPPER AND LOWER BODY EXERCISES 89

CHAPTER 10: CHAIR YOGA FOR STRENGTH AND MOBILITY 235

CONCLUSION 255

Introduction

What would you do to reverse the signs and symptoms of aging? What would you do to stay strong, active, and independent as you get older? We have been fascinated for centuries by the idea of remaining youthful or delaying the effects of aging. The Spanish explorer, Ponce de León, searched endlessly for the mythical fountain of youth in the 16th century, but instead discovered Florida. Oscar Wilde's Dorian Gray relegated his aging to a portrait, which, in the end, didn't work out so well for him. But I think Mark Twain captured it best when he said, "Life would be infinitely better if we could only be born at the age of 80 and gradually approach 18."

I can't say whether or not the fountain of youth exists and I'm fairly certain we can't consign our aging to a portrait, but that doesn't mean we can't find a way to not only increase our longevity, but to increase our quality of life and simultaneously delay the onset of aging. While we may not be able to altogether stop the process of aging)which is mostly determined by our genetics and therefore unchangeable) we can control other factors in our lives that speed up the process like stress, lifestyle habits, and physical activity.

The best way to reverse the aging process is by taking care of our bodies through better nutrition and regular exercise, particularly strength training. By concentrating on those things you can control, you can end up younger biologically than you are chronologically. This translates into not only living longer, but feeling better and doing the things you enjoy for a much longer time.

In our youth, we tend to spend a lot of time focusing on what we eat and getting at least some exercise. As we get older, however, we start to pay less attention to our bodies and our health. We know life and responsibilities are more important as we get older and we often let our own health and wellness get shuffled to the sidelines. Sooner or later we wake up, as older adults, with stiffness in our joints and trouble moving. Daily tasks seem like an effort and we find ourselves in our doctor's office, only to learn that we have diabetes or hypertension.

I walked out of my doctor's office more than 15 years ago with the knowledge that I was now diabetic. I was shocked and dazed to say the least, but it also made me realize that I needed to do things differently and take control of the situation. If I continued as I was, I would be dependent on my sons sooner than I wanted to be, and I would no longer be able to enjoy the life I currently had. So I chose to change my eating and exercise habits. As a result, I've spent the last 15 years finding the best and most practical exercises to manage my disease and to live independently. I know what it's like to get older and be affected by illness and feel like you're losing control. But I also know what it feels like to find a way forward again and make the changes that can delay the aging process, as well as make you feel younger and healthier. This book is a testament to that journey of discovery, and I'm sharing it with you so that you, too, can choose to lead a different, more active life, and defy the aging odds.

It doesn't matter if you're already physically active or if you've never done a workout a day in your life, as this book will be your guide to finding the right strength exercises and the right mindset to build your muscles, strengthen your body, and increase your mobility and flexibility. Strengthening the muscles around your joints, particularly those of your hips and knees, will increase your mobility and reduce your risk of falling and unsteadiness.

What to Expect

It is never too late to start exercising, even if you consider yourself a senior. There is, in fact, a lot of debate over what is considered "senior" because a 65-year old senior is obviously very different from a 90-year old senior. The point here is, regardless of your age or your level of fitness, anyone can build muscle and get stronger. Regular exercise and strength training as an older adult can help you avoid muscle loss as you get older and ensure that you maintain your strength and independence.

As we age, we may experience reduced mobility, changes in vision, loss of muscle mass, digestive issues, and changes in brain function. Most of these issues can be reversed with a more active lifestyle. The Centers for Disease Control (CDC) recommends that older adults get at least 30 minutes of moderate physical activity five days a week (2019). Two of those days should include strength training, and at least three days should have a balance and flexibility element. The idea is to move more and sit less.

The more sedentary your lifestyle, the greater your loss of muscles, balance, and mobility, which can lead to a higher risk of falling and injury. The CDC estimates that an older adult suffers from a fall every second in the United States. That's about 36 million falls each year and accounts for about 32,000 deaths (2021). The best way to stay safe and maintain your independence is to get moving.

I can assure you that your life will be so much easier once you make exercising a part of your daily routine. Playing with your grandkids, carrying your groceries into the house, getting in and out of a chair, reaching items on a shelf, and other daily tasks will all be easier when you're stronger, not just physically, but mentally and emotionally. If you can move easily and do your chores independently because you are stronger, it will boost your confidence and can fight feelings of anxiety and depression.

We will first explore how aging works and the factors that contribute to it. You will better understand the parts of aging you can and cannot control, and how they can impact the rate at which you age. I will share tips guaranteed to slow down the aging process and help you lead a fuller, stronger life.

Remember: Stronger means not only our bodies but our minds. Before we delve into our physical exercise routines, we will devote some time to our mental and emotional wellness. We know that aging affects our brain function, but more than that, aging can affect how we view ourselves and our bodies. In addition to a physical effect, getting older impacts us on a psychological level and we worry about our ability to remain self-sufficient. We stress over day-to-day tasks and sometimes we feel alone. Before we can dedicate ourselves to a daily physical routine, we need to encourage and grow our mental strength. Without a strong, confident mind, your body may not have the willpower to commit to maintaining a strong body.

Once you begin to foster that mental strength, you can work to create the space and mood for physical activity. Just as we took the time to understand the aging process and to focus on our mental health, we need to learn how to best prepare our bodies for physical activity. This is particularly important as an older adult because we want to ensure that we are doing an activity that is right for our physical abilities, our fitness level, and our mental readiness. We want to find the best way to motivate ourselves to make exercise part of our daily routine. To establish this connection, we have to learn the proper warm-up techniques (to avoid injuries), how to breathe (efficiently and steadily) while exercising, and what music can motivate us, along with how to adjust it based on the exercise we are doing.

When you begin an exercise routine, especially if you've led a fairly sedentary lifestyle up to this point, you may find it difficult to perform some of the exercises. In fact, you may already be experiencing pain and stiffness when getting up or doing daily tasks. But don't be disheartened. The more you move, the more you will strengthen and lengthen the muscles in your body, thereby improving your mobility and your flexibility. This means you can move more easily and do your chores without any help or fear of injury. Greater mobility will boost your confidence and leave you feeling accomplished.

Once you've started moving and you gain confidence in your abilities, you will want to start focusing on specific exercises that strengthen your upper and lower body. Do you have trouble opening a jar or picking up your grandkids? It's probably because the muscles in your arms and legs are weakening primarily due to age and lack of use. A lack of exercise can cause some muscles to tighten and others to loosen, leading to an imbalance which can, in turn, lead to pain and problems moving. Working to strengthen these key areas ensures your continued independence and delays the effects of aging on your body. Again, you can build and strengthen muscle at any age. So, the more you use those muscles, the more you will gain.

The joints in our hips and knees carry the majority of our weight and therefore are more prone to wear and tear. As we age, we are more susceptible to pain and inflammation in these joints. A regular exercise routine and daily physical activity can help reduce pain and discomfort in your joints. Exercising daily can help you maintain your weight while strengthening and stretching the muscles around your joints. This means you can feel sure in your movements as you go about your daily activities.

Adding some low impact cardio to your routine is an excellent way to get the blood flowing and your heart rate up, and the great thing is that you can do it no matter your level of fitness. A cardio routine increases the strength in your muscles, bones, lungs, and heart, thereby increasing your mobility. This means daily movement becomes easier, and you experience less stiffness in your joints.

As you strengthen the muscles in your upper and lower body, it is vital that you pay attention to the muscles that make up your core. Without a strong core, you won't be able to do even the simplest of tasks. A strong core is necessary for the overall strength of your body and is responsible for balance, stability, and good posture. A strong core facilitates a broader range of motion which means that your daily activities won't feel like too much effort, and you will have more energy. All of these effects together will boost your confidence and reduce your risk of falling and injury.

Building strength, particularly as we age, is vital for ensuring our continued independence. That being said, sometimes we want a routine that not only strengthens our bodies, but nourishes and calms our minds. A total body yoga routine is a superb way to attain all the benefits of a strength workout while paying attention to your emotional and mental needs. The yoga routine here is specifically designed for older adults to help you build your practice, focus on how you breathe while building and strengthening your muscles, and increase your flexibility and mobility. You will find yourself developing more confidence in your abilities and performing your day-to-day routine with ease.

All the exercise routines you will find in this book have been carefully selected to meet the needs of older adults who want to continue to lead independent and healthy lives. They have helped me through my daily tasks, as well as those that require more of me. I want the same for you as you enter the prime of your life. But before you begin (as I know you're eager to!), take a few moments to read about some of the things you will need, as well as a few tips to ensure that you are safe while becoming stronger.

What You Need

As with any physical activity, it is important that you speak with your doctor or other healthcare professional before beginning. The exercise routines in this book have been created with seniors in mind, so there is minimum impact on your joints, and modifications have been made to take into account balance and mobility issues. It is, however, still advisable to get the go-ahead from your doctor.

For these workouts, you will need a chair (preferably without a padded seat) with a straight back and no arms, and if possible, a set of two-pound hand weights and a mat for floor exercises. Be sure to wear loose, comfortable clothing that will keep you cool and is easy to move in. Restrictive clothing can make you uncomfortable during exercise and can affect your willingness to continue the activity. Be sure to wear appropriate footwear that fits well and is comfortable.

If you're practicing on tiles, be careful that they are not slippery.

A huge motivational factor for a workout is finding a space that works for you and that you will enjoy returning to on a daily basis. Ensure that the space you choose is large enough for your chair or mat, and that you can fully extend your arms and legs. When selecting or creating your space, let it be a reflection of you and your personality. The space should motivate you to want to do your activity. Try not to have too much clutter; it will distract. If you're practicing with a group of friends, work together to create a space that all of you can enjoy and get the encouragement you need, in order to commit to your daily physical activity.

Once you've found that perfect spot, try to find the time of day that works best for you. If you're just starting out, experiment with different times and observe how you feel before and after your workout. A morning workout can give you consistently better sleep and reduce your feelings of hunger, while doing your workout in the afternoon means your body is already warmed up and your cortisol (stress hormone) levels are lower (as they usually peak in the morning). Afternoon exercise may, however, disrupt your circadian rhythm. Regardless of what time you choose, try to be consistent. Consistency helps you to create a routine for your body and mind.

If you have never exercised, or haven't for a long time, it is probably best to start with fewer repetitions and sets, and then work your way up to more as you get stronger and more confident. Importantly, make sure that you are hydrated before and after your practice. Above all else, relax and have fun.

Safety Tips

You're probably eager to jump right into a begin exercising, but here are a few things you should consider before you begin:

Make an appointment with your doctor.

Any change to your daily routine, especially when it involves physical activity, should be discussed with your primary healthcare provider. They will know best what you should and should not do, and you can work together to come up with the best plan to suit your individual needs.

1. **Follow the instructions.**

    The exercise instructions are created with older adults in mind. There are modifications already built-in to cater for fitness and mobility levels. Altering the exercise can result in serious injury, so be sure to follow closely. If anything feels uncomfortable, then stop the activity and talk to your doctor.

2. **Start slow and don't overdo it.**

   Building strength and increasing muscle mass takes time and patience. The routine you choose should challenge you, but should not be overwhelming. Doing an activity that is not at your level can lead to injuries. If you find that you cannot complete a routine, then you may want to consider reducing the intensity and the number of repetitions.

3. **Warm up properly.**

   A warm-up routine is an essential part of your workout. You need to give your body the opportunity to adjust. Warming up and stretching will ensure that your muscles are not sore at the end of your activity, and it will significantly reduce the chances of injury.

4. **Always stay hydrated.**

   Dehydration is a concern for older adults in general, but becomes even more critical when you're exercising. If you don't get enough fluids, you can experience headaches, muscle cramps, weakness, and dizziness, all of which can lead to injury.

Each chapter of this book will guide you through exercises targeting various parts of your body. Once you're comfortable with the movements, you can mix and match them to suit your needs. However, always be certain to begin with the warm-up routine. If any exercise doesn't feel right, or if you feel any pain or discomfort, stop doing the exercise, and talk to your doctor. This is the beginning of your journey to better health and reversing the signs of aging.

Chapter 1:

Understanding Aging and What You Can Do to Slow It Down

As we get older, we begin to notice more gray hairs, along with wrinkles, then we start experiencing pain in our back and joints, as well as muscle stiffness when we wake up in the morning or when we perform certain tasks. When we experience these symptoms, we tend to believe that we should do less and move less—basically, we should stop doing and enjoying the things we love. But we need to take a moment to understand the process of aging and how it works, as well as what we can do to age differently, or even better.

Aging does not have to mean the end of our independence or enjoyment of life. If we recognize what our bodies need, then getting older can definitely be a joyful experience. Treating our bodies well, choosing healthy foods, making better lifestyle choices, getting regular check-ups, and most importantly, staying physically active are the best ways to slow down and maybe even reverse the aging process.

The Aging Process

Aging is an inevitable part of life, and as we age, our bodies change, making us feel different and move differently. The structures and functions of our cells decline over time but we can delay the process of aging, as well as the symptoms that come with getting older.

Aging can fall into two categories:

1. Intrinsic

2. Extrinsic

Intrinsic aging is genetically predetermined and part of the natural process of our cells. Cells are programmed to divide, multiply, and perform various biological functions but the more they divide, the older they become. Young cells are able to repair themselves quickly and with minimal effort. As cells age, they begin to lose their ability to function properly, increasing the time it takes for cells to repair. As such, cellular damage increases. Older cells, therefore, are less healthy.

For instance, when we are younger, our skin is smoother and more elastic because our skin cells are younger and can quickly repair or replace any damaged cells. As we age, the replacement of these cells slows and this can be seen in the appearance of wrinkles, decreased elasticity, and overall dryness of our skin.

Similarly, muscle cells are self-renewing, even as we get older. However, the less we use our muscles, the quicker they weaken as we age. The right lifestyle choices can delay the loss of muscle function. These include adding more aerobic exercises into our daily routine, such as walking and swimming, doing resistance and bodyweight training, increasing other activities like yoga, stretching, and core work to our routines, and increasing our consumption of protein.

Extrinsic aging relates to external or environmental factors over which we may have a bit more control. These include where we live, our levels of stress, and our lifestyle. It also encompasses air pollution, tobacco use, alcohol consumption, and malnutrition. Most of these are elements we can control and adjust, in order to slow down the aging process.

Our age is a combination of our chronological as well as our biological age. Like intrinsic aging, we have little control over our chronological age—the number will change every year no matter what. However, our biological age is determined by our level of fitness, our mental awareness, and our overall health and wellness. Much like extrinsic aging, our biological age can be influenced by our food choices, our exercise routine, our lifestyle decisions, and even our social activity. In some instances, our biological age can be impacted by our genetics. We could be more genetically predisposed to illness or diseases—this we cannot control.

We should, however, work on the things we can control and change. Aging doesn't have to be associated with frailty and dependency. In the past, we tended to place everyone over the age of 65 in the same category, but we really cannot do that anymore. You cannot compare a 65-year old adult to an 85-year old adult. They differ in their physical abilities, their muscle strength, their recovery time, and even in their cognitive function.

Increased life expectancy because of better nutrition and hygiene, as well as access to healthcare and improvements in modern medicine, means that we are living longer lives. So, a 65-year old in good health cannot be considered or treated in the same way as an 85-year old. Chances are that we may still be both independent and active, but to varying degrees. All these factors must be taken into consideration as we seek to understand the aging process in light of all the physical, environmental, and scientific factors.

Habits to Avoid

Now, we know that there are some things we can't control when it comes to aging, but there are also things—particular habits—we can change to slow down the aging process. Of course, some habits, like brushing your teeth and washing your hands, are beneficial and should be done, but there are others that can be harmful and even affect how quickly you age.

Unhealthy Food

We all know that eating a nutritious and well-balanced diet is key to staying healthy and living a longer life, but many older adults opt for foods that feel comfortable and familiar. These foods tend to be high in carbohydrates and calories but lacking in most other nutrients. Eating your fruits and vegetables can go a long way in delaying the process and signs of aging.

Fruits and vegetables contain the nutrients you need to repair damaged cells and protect them from further harm. The nutrients in these foods also reduce your risk of heart disease. Avoid 'diet' foods and those that are highly processed and instead opt for whole foods like fresh fruits and vegetables. Also, try to abstain from snacking late at night because more likely than not, you will pick an unhealthy snack that is high in calories but low in nutritional value.

Inactivity

As we get older, we sometimes have a tendency to move less, and the less we move the more likely we are to experience pain and stiffness. A sedentary lifestyle, particularly for an older adult, can increase your risk of obesity, heart disease, diabetes, and stroke. A lack of movement also contributes to muscle loss, which can affect your balance and stability, making you more susceptible to falling.

Staying active can go a long way in maintaining strength in your muscles and giving you the confidence you need to go about your daily activities. Being active also means that you can hold on to your independence for a longer time. Remember, our chronological age is not the only determinant of our age. Our biological age plays a huge part in how we look and feel and move. By exercising, we can positively affect our biological age which contributes to our overall health and wellness.

Smoking

Harmful habits we start in our youth are oftentimes difficult to break when we are older—smoking is one of those habits. Cigarettes and related tobacco products contain toxins that can affect your organs, particularly your largest organ—your skin. Smoking can lead to premature aging and wrinkles, as well as narrowing your blood vessels, thereby restricting the flow of blood and oxygen to other parts of your body.

Tobacco smoke damages the cells in your body so rapidly that the cells are never able to repair themselves or regenerate quickly enough to replace the damaged ones. This speeds up the rate at which we appear to age, causing deep wrinkles and sagging skin. This premature aging caused by smoking can also affect your mental health, leading you to periods of sadness and depression. If you are exercising, tobacco smoke can also affect your performance and stamina.

Ideally, it would be best to avoid tobacco altogether, but if you do smoke, you should consider the health implications and try to reduce your usage. Talk to your healthcare provider about finding a way that works best for you to lower or eliminate your tobacco intake. It will take time, but in the long-term, it will be worth it to have a longer, healthier, independent life.

Alcohol

Like tobacco use, your alcohol consumption should be limited or lowered. Alcohol can diminish cognitive function, weaken your organs, dehydrate your skin, affect your heart, lower your immune response, and even impact your medication. Furthermore, it can affect your balance. Older adults are already at a higher risk of falling, and consuming alcohol only heightens that risk.

Alcohol consumption can also worsen diseases like osteoporosis, diabetes, and high blood pressure—all of which contribute to aging and ill health. This is because alcohol, like tobacco, affects our cells' ability to heal and regenerate themselves. It effectively slows down or sometimes destroys the cells' recovery process. This means that not only do we age more quickly, we are also more likely to suffer from illness and diseases.

Moreover, alcohol can prevent you from sustaining habits that keep you healthy and free from illness. Because alcohol can make you feel listless, you are less likely to want to be active. For an older adult, as we know, inactivity can be dangerous. It can lead to weight gain, diabetes, inflammation, and pain, all of which can cause you to age rapidly. Alcohol also damages your brain cells, and these cannot be replaced once they're damaged, which means it can affect your cognitive function. If you do want to have a drink, consider having no more than one per day, but be sure to talk to your doctor to make sure that it won't affect any of your medications.

Skipping Regular Checkups

I know going to the doctor is never anyone's favorite task, but as we get older, it's no longer a simple item to check off our list—it's a necessity. There is a greater risk of health complications as we get older and sometimes there are no symptoms until the illness has gotten worse. Getting regular checkups from your primary care physician, provides them the chance to better detect and treat any possible issues that may rise. This gives you a better chance of continuing to live a healthy, independent life.

As you get older, a regular health screening should include an eye and hearing exam, blood sugar and blood pressure checks, vaccination updates, dementia and depression checks, as well as height and weight checks. Your risk of falling may also be assessed. Men may also have a prostate exam, while women should have a pap smear and mammogram done.

It may seem like a lot, but regular visits to your doctor are definitely worthwhile. You can work with your doctor to manage any chronic conditions you may have and create a diet and exercise plan that will ensure that you can continue to be self-sufficient for as long as possible. Your doctor is trained to identify what symptoms mean and how they can be treated. So the next time your annual checkup comes around, make sure you go.

Ignoring Your Family History

When we're young, we think we're invincible, and the illnesses of our parents and grandparents are not relevant to us. As we age, though, we realize that our family health history plays a major role in our health and aging.

Knowledge of your family health history can help you to determine if you are at a higher risk for any diseases, including high blood pressure, diabetes, stroke, and certain forms of cancer. Knowing your family history can allow you to take the necessary steps to reduce your own risk for these diseases, many times through lifestyle or environmental changes. It's important to share your family health history with your healthcare provider. They can help you to determine what you need to do or what preventative steps you may need to take.

Having a family history of a particular disease or illness does not necessarily mean that you will also have it, but it is always better to be aware and prepared to take the necessary steps to deal with it. Knowing about your family history is only half of it. You must act on it in order to prevent any potential illness. Part of acting is making sure you have your regular checkups, stay active, and eat well while making healthy lifestyle choices.

Habits are sometimes difficult to break and it takes time to change habits. The key is to remain consistent and find a way that works best for you without being stressful. Avoiding the habits we've just discussed can go a long way in slowing down the aging process and allow you to live a healthier, fuller, and more independent life.

Exercising to Stay Young

We've all heard that we should exercise to stay healthy, fit, and young, but how does exercising really make a difference as we age? When we're younger, our motivation to exercise primarily stems from our desire to look a certain way, but as we age, exercise should become a part of our daily routine. The more sedentary our lifestyle is as we get older, the greater our chances of hospitalization and doctor's visits. It also means that you may need to increase your medications, and you won't be able to continue doing the things you love.

When we're inactive for too long, our bodies become unaccustomed to movement, so when we do have to move, it requires more effort and energy. This, in turn, makes us tired and short of breath quickly, even after the simplest task. If we remain active as we get older, we can maintain our body's ability to efficiently use energy. As a result, our quality of life is better and we are capable of moving around easily.

In many instances, the condition of our skin can make us look older because of the appearance of fine lines and wrinkles. Exercise can actually help to keep your skin looking younger. When you are physically active, you increase blood flow in your body, which means that more oxygen is being transported to your cells. This, then, results in healthier cells. The increased blood flow nourishes your cells and the more oxygen the cells receive, the better able they are to rid themselves of waste. In fact, when we sweat, our pores open and release any waste build up. Sweat purges the toxins from our body, leaving our skin cells healthier and more oxygenated. So instead of heading to the drugstore for some anti-aging moisturizer, try adding at least 30 minutes of exercise to your daily routine.

As we know, muscle loss and changes to our bone density are part of the aging process and as a result, there is a decline in our healthy posture. Fortunately, we can prevent and even reverse the loss of muscle, along with the weakening of our bones. Exercising, particularly strength training, can work to rebuild your muscles, as well as prevent any further bone loss. It also helps you to maintain a strong body and strong joints. Subsequently, exercise leaves you with a taller, straighter posture that keeps you looking and feeling younger. Stronger bones and more muscle also decreases your risk of falling and of injury, which means you can be more assured in your movements as you perform your daily tasks.

Furthermore, exercise increases your flexibility. When we are inactive, our muscles and joints can become stiff and difficult to move. This makes tasks, like getting up from a chair or lifting groceries, increasingly difficult. By exercising, you increase the flexibility of your muscles and lubricate your joints, which reduces your chance of injury (particularly hip injuries) and increases the likelihood of living a longer, healthier life.

As our age goes up, our metabolism goes down, and not exercising makes the decline quicker. A slower metabolism means that we are more likely to gain weight, which then puts us at an increased risk for illnesses, such as type 2 diabetes and heart disease. Regular physical activity can increase our muscle mass, which then increases our metabolism, allowing us to burn more calories. We are, therefore, better able to maintain a steady, healthy weight and lower our chances of illness if we workout regularly.

Just as our bodies are important as we age, so is our mind. Like our muscles, if we don't make regular use of our brain, it will decline. Our hippocampus is the region of our brain that controls learning and memory. If the cells in this area are not used, they will eventually die, and as we already know, brain cells cannot be replaced. Regular exercise increases the size of our hippocampus and encourages the health and survival of our brain cells. By exercising, you will truly have the brain of a younger person, and your mental acuity will be intact for many, many years.

We've all heard that stress can age us quickly. As we get older, we tend to have more stress in our lives and sometimes our stress stems from the actual process of aging. Stress can affect our longevity, as well as our ability to focus on and complete day-to-day tasks. Exercise increases the endorphins in our body that make us feel good and reduce our cortisol (stress hormone) levels. Daily exercise can boost our mood and help us manage our stress levels, allowing us to live longer lives and delay the aging process.

The bottom line is that strong muscles, bones, and joints keep us mobile and stable, and the only way to ensure that we stay strong is through regular exercise.

Daily physical activity will aid us in achieving our ultimate goal as we get older—maintaining our independence. Increased blood flow, a better range of motion, reduced muscle stiffness and back pain, healthier posture and alignment, and more efficient movement in general, are all steps toward continued self-sufficiency. None of this will be possible if we don't commit ourselves to moving regularly.

Aging Without Injury

Falls and other accidents become more common as we age and can result in serious injuries, including hip fractures, traumatic brain injuries, and other permanent disabilities. More than one in four older adults report falling each year—that's about 36 million falls (Centers for Disease Control, 2021). Fortunately, there are steps we can take to prevent us from falling and avoid risk of injury.

One of your first steps should be to talk with your physician at your next checkup. If you're feeling unsteady when you stand or walk, or if you have any doubts about your movement or range of motion, discuss these things with your doctor. Also, make sure you review any medications that you may be taking with your doctor as well. The way in which medications work or affect us may change as we get older. Some may cause dizziness or make you feel unstable. Your primary healthcare provider will know what to do or if you need to change your medication. It may also be a good idea to chat with them about taking vitamin D, if you're not already. Vitamin D, particularly as we age, is vital for bone, muscle, and nerve health.

At your yearly medical visit, you should also have your eyes checked. Healthy eyes and good vision go a long way in preventing falls and accidents. Your doctor should check for cataract or glaucoma as well. If you're having problems with your vision, don't wait to have your eyes examined. It may mean the difference between continued independence and a serious injury.

At that same annual visit, have your feet checked. It may seem like it's unnecessary, but our feet are responsible for keeping us standing and bearing all of our weight. If your feet hurt regularly or you experience pain or discomfort when standing, you should mention this to your doctor. Many times, we simply aren't wearing the appropriate footwear. As we get older, our feet require the proper support and cushioning and they need to be taken care of like the rest of our body.

At these visits, your physician will also tell you that it's important that you stay active, as this is the best way to prevent falls and injuries. Aging weakens our muscles and increases our chances of falling. To counteract the effects of aging, focus on engaging in regular physical activities, particularly ones that strengthen your lower body and legs. Chat with your healthcare provider to find the program that would work best for you and suit your needs.

Your physical wellness is only part of the solution to avoiding injuries. The other part is making your home safer, especially if you live on your own. Even if we are physically fit, small things in our homes can lead to falls. You should remove anything that could be considered a trip hazard, such as small throw rugs and mats, on which you can easily stumble. Keeping your floors free of clutter is an easy way to prevent a fall.

Even if your vision is good, it is always useful to add more or brighter lights to your home, making it easier to see and identify any potential hazards. You should even consider leaving a light on at night if you tend to wake up to use the bathroom. In your bathroom, you should add grab bars near your tub and toilet to assist you when getting up. They have really attractive options now that won't stand out if you're concerned about aesthetics. You should also consider adding handrails on both sides of your steps for additional support and balance.

Aging does not mean that you have to stop doing the things you love, or that you can no longer live independently. It simply means that you need to take a few extra precautions to ensure that you can continue to do all those things for a long time to come, without needing any help.

It's Never Too Late to Start Living a Healthy Life

So, you've gotten all this information about aging and how to delay it, but you've never really led an active or especially healthy lifestyle before, or maybe you stopped a long time ago. In that case, will it really make a difference now if you exercise and make better choices? The answer is, most emphatically, YES!

Physical activity and healthy lifestyle choices can be beneficial no matter what age you are or when you start. Meeting that recommended weekly goal of 150 minutes can seem a bit daunting when you're starting out, but it is doable, and the routines in this book will help you to get there.

Exercising should include aerobic activity, as well as strength training and balance and flexibility exercises. Even if you've been mostly sedentary, doing them now can reduce your mortality risk and reverse some of the effects of aging.

You don't need to be a super athlete to reap the rewards of daily physical activity. You will sleep better, feel better, and function better. You will also reduce your chances of a host of illnesses including heart disease, stroke, hypertension, type 2 diabetes, depression, certain types of cancer, and, of course, falls. Through exercising, you can even reverse the effects on your heart caused by sedentary aging. Exercising increases the elasticity of your heart muscles, reducing cardiac stiffness, thereby lowering your risk for heart complications.

So even if you've never exercised as a young adult, consider doing so now. Living a sedentary life will only make you age faster and keep you from doing the things you want to do. Adding just a little bit of exercise to your day and making some healthier choices can mean the difference between dependency and self-sufficiency as you get older.

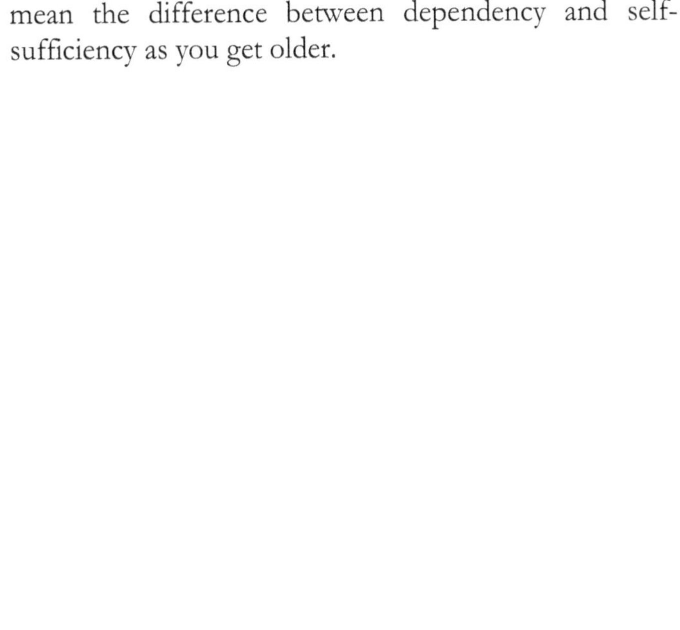

Chapter 2:

Strengthening Our Minds

to Strengthen Our Bodies

The decision to be active and to make better lifestyle choices is a physical decision as much as it is a psychological and mental decision. For us to commit to strengthening our bodies, we must have the will and mental fortitude to stick with it and make it work for us. Our mental health and wellness, likewise, is as important as our physical well-being.

Our mental health refers to our psychological and emotional state of mind, and influences how we perceive or react to various experiences, as well as how we feel physically and emotionally. A strong body requires a strong mind, and to keep our minds active, we need to move.

As we age, the state of our mental health becomes even more crucial and can affect our overall well-being. Good mental health gives us the energy we need to manage and deal with our daily tasks and stress. It encourages us to socialize with our peers and to participate in group and social activities. Mental health wellness can be the difference between productivity and dependency.

For the last two and a half years, we have been in the throes of the COVID-19pandemic and it has taken a toll on all of us. Particularly during the early days of the pandemic, seniors bore the brunt of the measures aimed at reducing the spread of the virus. They have faced, and continue to face severe restrictions to in-person gatherings, travel, visitations, recreation, and entertainment. During lockdowns, they have even had to resort to tele-medicine for checkups out of fear for what could happen if they had an in-person visit.

As a result of these drastic measures, older adults were cut off from their social networks that normally provided emotional support during difficult times. These social networks were important for older adults to have the chance to express themselves and engage with others. As a result, the social distancing measures put in place were akin to social isolation, increasing the feelings of loneliness experienced by seniors. This social isolation translated into a reduction in the quality of life for older adults and an increased risk of premature death, stroke, and dementia. The loneliness associated with the pandemic increased instances of anxiety and emotional instability among older adults, as well as cases of hypertension, inflammation, and high levels of stress hormones (Webb and Chen, 2021).

Finding Our Mental Strength

As we emerge from this pandemic, we begin to find ways to return to a certain normalcy that can allow us to be with others, as well as have that feeling of companionship. Our brain likes to be challenged and being in a social setting can engage various cognitive systems like speaking, remembering, and learning, and helps alleviate the loneliness and isolation we may have felt during the most restrictive periods of lockdown.

We are generally social beings, and as we age, our need for camaraderie deepens. Finding ways to exercise and engage our brain can improve our cognitive skills. Brain exercises can be imaginative or tactile. Imaginative activities emphasize focus, attention, and problem solving skills, while our tactile exercises stimulate different types of memory skills.

Part of our mental health includes our brain health. This involves ensuring that our brain functions optimally at a biological, behavioral, and subjective level. As I mentioned before, our brain health is connected to our physical health. The more we move, the more we reduce our risk of cognitive impairment and increase our cognitive function.

Physical activity increases our heart rate, which in turn increases the flow of blood to our cells. As a result, more oxygen is transported to our brain, triggering the release of hormones that stimulate the growth of new connections between our brain cells associated with executive function and memory. This is critical, considering our executive function controls our emotions, helps us to regulate our behavior and responses to situations, and allows us to plan and organize our daily tasks. As you get older, preserving and strengthening our executive function becomes essential to maintaining our independence.

Furthermore, the boost in blood flow because of exercise increases the release of chemicals that aid in the communication between neurons, which means that our memory and our cognitive abilities can stay sharper for longer. Physical activity along with mental stimulation can delay the effects of aging while making us psychologically, emotionally, and mentally stronger.

In the chapters to follow, I will be sharing many workout routines to help make you strong physically and promote brain health, but before we embark on those exercises, I want to share with you a few activities to get you started on your mental health and wellness.

Cognitive Activities for Older Adults

1. **Crossword Puzzles**

    When doing crosswords puzzles, you need to use verbal memory to search for specific words that correlate to the clue. This engages the brain in memory recall and may possibly aid in delaying the onset of memory decline in persons with dementia.

2. **Online Brain Games**

    Games like Luminosity and Brain HQ challenge your memory, attention, and concentration. Challenging your brain in this way creates and strengthens the neural pathways associated with these functions.

3. Building Models

When we have to follow detailed instructions and put pieces together in a certain way, it helps with procedural memory, as well as the brain functions connected to understanding, remembering, and performing a task.

4. Jigsaw Puzzles

Puzzles are always a great way to relax and spend some time in the company of others while doing something together. More significantly, building puzzles strengthens your visual-spatial working memory, which simply means your ability to see and remember which pieces go where, in order to complete the puzzle.

5. Physical Activity

Activities like walking, swimming, yoga, and strength training are physical activities, but they play a major role in cognitive health. Exercise increases cell production in the hippocampus, the region of the brain responsible for memory, learning, and emotions. The hippocampus is unique because it is the only part of the brain where new cells can be made. Therefore, physical activity plays a role in boosting and maintaining our memory and learning, as well as helping us to manage our emotional well-being.

Our mental health is as important as our physical health and being physically healthy can promote better mental wellness. It is important for us to understand what happens to us psychologically and emotionally as we get older and to take the steps to ensure that we are nourishing our mind, body, and spirit. As you progress through the physical routines in this book, take a few moments at the start and the end to check in with yourself psychologically and emotionally, and know that by dedicating time to exercising, you are fortifying yourself mentally too.

Chapter 3:

Why Breathing, Stretching, and Music Are So Important

Better Breathing for Greater Endurance

We all know how to breathe. It's a pretty standard part of our day-to-day lives and doesn't require any instructions, right? This is true for the most part, but there may be a more efficient way to breathe, particularly when you're exercising.

The more you move, the more oxygen your muscles will require. The idea behind breathing more efficiently is to allow more oxygen to be delivered, which in turn makes your muscles work better.

As we age, our lung capacity diminishes, making us more susceptible to respiratory ailments. The size of our bones is reduced and our rib cage loses mobility, which means there is less room for our lungs to expand. Muscles, like the diaphragm, weaken over time, and as a result, the volume of air we exhale is lower. Subsequently, there is less room for new oxygen to enter our bodies, and the level of carbon dioxide in our bodies rises, leading to fatigue and shortness of breath.

Frequent exercise can increase and maintain our lung capacity, but it is critical that we practice proper breathing. It is usually best to breathe in and out through your nose, since your nose acts as your body's natural air filter. It can warm or cool the air as needed and protect you against millions of foreign particles circulating in the air. More relevant is the fact that breathing through your nose reduces the rate of exertion during exercise and daily activities. This means that you will feel less tired during and after an activity if you breathe through your nose.

Moreover, the way in which we breathe sends signals to our brain. Breathing through your nose lowers your nervous system's 'fight or flight' response to any situation. Breathing deeply and focusing on your breath can decrease cortisol (hormones responsible for stress) levels. It can also help to reduce your feelings of depression and anxiety. Proper breathing practice may stabilize as well as lower your blood pressure levels while strengthening your core and can also offset insomnia and sleeplessness.

The best way to breathe is diaphragmatically. This means taking slow, deep breaths that fill up your abdominal area as opposed to just your chest. Most of us take shallow breaths that fill our chest area but never quite reach our bellies. By breathing from our diaphragm, we activate the muscles in our core and allow for more oxygen to enter our bodies. This, in turn, helps us avoid stitches and cramps in our sides when we're exercising. Also, breathing in and out through our noses slows our rate of breathing and requires less exertion, helping us to maintain a steadier and more even breath during physical activities.

When you're performing strength exercises, you should breathe out when you lift an object and out as you lower it. Breathing out as you lift increases the engagement of your core muscles and prevents your blood pressure from dropping drastically. When doing mobility exercises, you should focus on long inhales and exhales. This will help with your range of motion, allowing you to go further and deeper into your movement. If you hold your breath, you will end up being tense and locking your muscles. Breathing helps to release that tension.

So, before you start any exercise, be sure to take at least three long deep breaths, focusing on filling up your belly. While you're exercising, keep returning to how you're breathing and try to keep your breaths slow and steady.

Warming-Up to Prepare

A warm-up is a gentle way to prepare your body for the rigors of your exercise routine. It helps to activate your muscles and should be specific to the muscles you plan to target during your workout. For instance, if you're planning to go for a run, then you should work on lower body stretches. Warming-up gives you an opportunity to mentally and physically prepare for the workout ahead of you, and should never be skipped. Your warm-up routine should be about 10 to 15 minutes long.

A warm-up routine usually includes some cardio work, some strength, and some stretching. Cardio helps to increase circulation and blood flow, as well as raise your body temperature and heart rate. Including strength activities in your warm-up allows you to gently increase your intensity level and prepares your body for sudden movements. Stretching, in turn, warms up your muscles and prepares your body in general for more vigorous movement. Tight muscles cannot go through their full range of motion if they are not warmed-up and activated.

In general, a thorough warm-up routine will increase the blood flow to your muscles, allowing for more access to oxygen. It steadily increases your body temperature and heart rate while improving your range of motion by stretching and lengthening your muscles, and will also loosen your joints. Most importantly, a proper warm-up will reduce your risk of injury during and after exercise. A warm-up also gives you the time to mentally prepare for the exertion required of you during your workout.

When you're stretching during your warm-up, be certain that you take it slowly and never stretch to the point of pain, as you'll end up doing more harm than good. As we've already noted, your breathing affects your heart rate and blood pressure, along with your nervous system. So, try to synchronize your breathing with your movements. Sometimes when we stretch, we tend to hold our breath. Make sure you're breathing slowly and deeply. Hold your stretches for between 20 and 30 seconds to give your muscles the time they need to lengthen. Above all else, do what feels right for you.

Music to Motivate

When you exercise, music can provide the ultimate adrenaline rush that will keep you moving. During low to moderate exercise, music actually boosts your energy levels, improves your mood, and delays the onset of exercise fatigue. If you listen to music prior to your workout, it can help to improve your performance during your tasks. Listening to music while you exercise can have activity-enhancing effects as well as psychological effects, allowing you to complete more repetitions or perform at a higher intensity. Music releases serotonin (a mood-boosting hormone) which makes you enjoy your workout, thereby keeping you moving.

Playing music while you exercise can even improve your coordination. The sounds increase the electrical activity in the parts of your brain responsible for coordinating movement. So, you may find yourself working out to the timing of the beat. This relationship between the auditory neurons (those related to sound) and the motor neurons (those concerned with movement) increases mental stimulation, which translates to enhanced exercise performance.

While an upbeat song will have you grooving through your workout, slow music at the end of your routine will lower your blood pressure and heart rate, as well as your recovery time. Slower music helps you to return more easily and quickly to your resting heart rate.

Perhaps one of the greatest benefits of music during your workout is that you focus more on the music than on the difficulty of the exercise and your feelings of tiredness. The music helps to shift your focus away from the physical sensations of your body (especially during lower-intensity workouts) and keeps you motivated. So, during your next workout, try some music and notice if it makes a difference to how you feel and how you perform. It's a great tool for focus and motivation.

Standing Warm-Up Routine

This is a comprehensive warm-up routine that will help your circulation and steadily increase your body temperature as you prepare for your workout. You can perform this routine before any of the exercises that follow. Make sure to take your time, pay attention to your breathing, and maybe put on some music to get you in the mood.

Neck Rotations

1. Stand straight with your feet hip-distance apart and your shoulders relaxed. Keep your arms at your sides.

2. Slowly turn your head to the right, then back to center, then to the left.

3. Repeat this movement until you have done three rotations on each side.

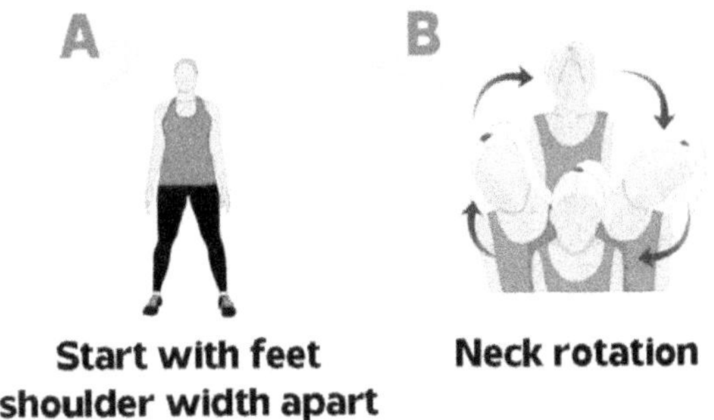

Start with feet shoulder width apart   **Neck rotation**

Neck Stretches

1. Begin by standing tall with your feet hip-distance apart and your arms relaxed down at your sides. Keep your shoulders away from your ears.

2. Gently lift your chin up toward the ceiling, then back to center. Following this, lower your chin down toward your chest, then return to center.

3. Perform this exercise three times in each direction.

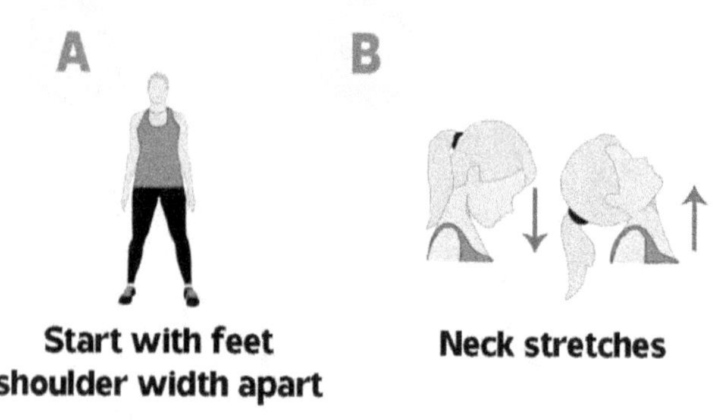

Start with feet shoulder width apart

Neck stretches

Shoulder Rolls

1. Stand with your feet hip-distance apart and your arms relaxed down at your sides.

2. Begin to make circles with your shoulders slowly in a clockwise direction.

3. Complete ten rolls in this direction, then switch and do ten more in the opposite direction.

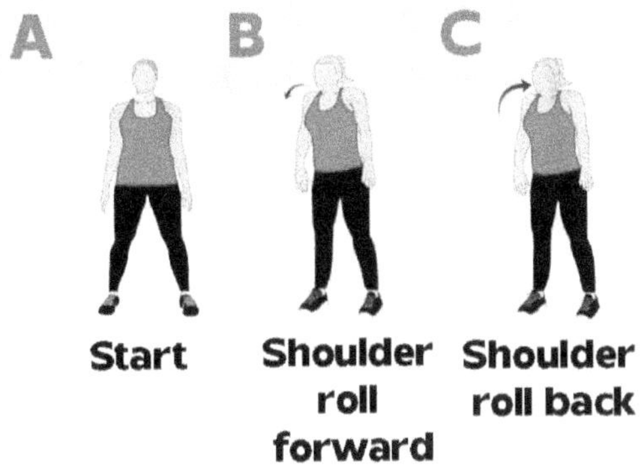

Arm Raises

1. Start by standing with your feet hip-width apart and your arms down along your sides.

2. Turn your hands so that your palms are facing inward and your thumbs are forward.

3. Slowly lift your arms forward, up, and over your head. Keep your shoulders away from your ears.

4. Then, slowly lower your arms back down to your starting position.

5. Repeat this movement three times.

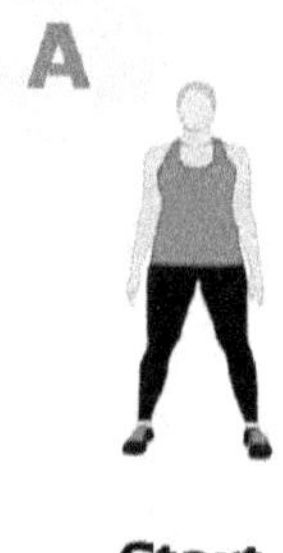

Start

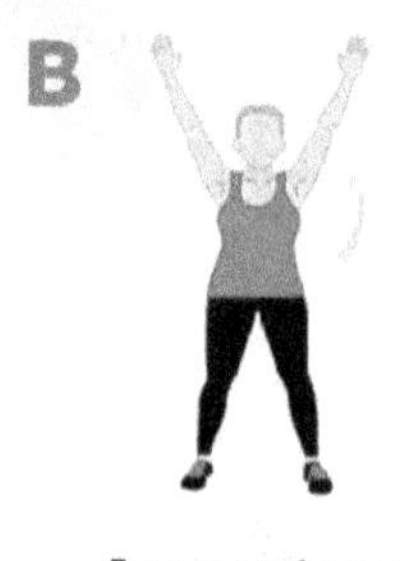

Arm raises

Toe Touch

1. Stand up tall with your feet hip-distance apart and your arms down at your sides, palms facing in.

2. Slowly lift your arms up over your head, then lean forward, lowering your arms and bending at your waist until you touch your toes (or as close as you can get).

3. Bend your knees and gently lift back up to your starting position with your arms at your sides.

4. Perform this exercise three times.

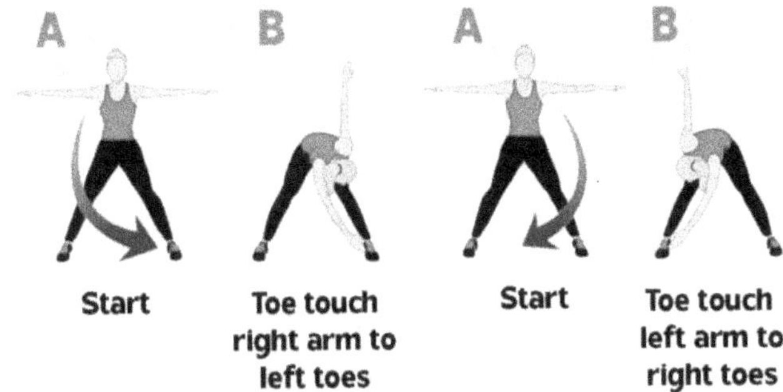

Knee Lift With Chair Support

1. Stand next to a chair with your feet hip-width apart and your toes pointing forward.

2. Place the hand closest to the chair on the chair back for support.

3. Lift your left knee up to about hip height (or as far as you can go) so that your leg is at a 90-degree angle, then gently lower it back down.

4. Now lift your right knee up to hip height and slowly lower it back.

5. Keep alternating between your left and right sides until you complete three repetitions on each side.

6. For more of a challenge, or if you have good balance, you can place your hands on your hips as you do these movements.

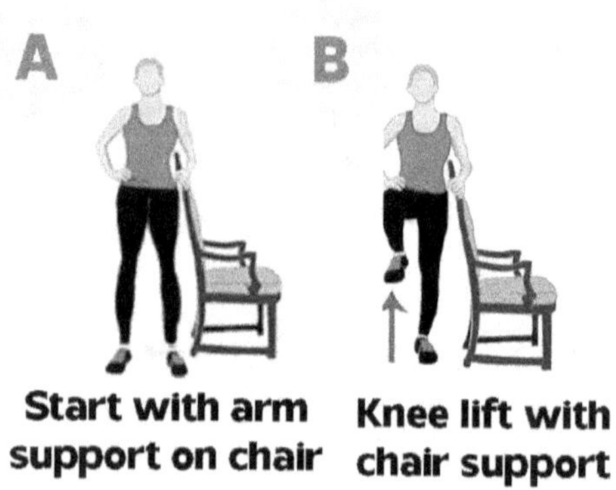

Start with arm support on chair   **Knee lift with chair support**

Shoulder Touch

1. Stand tall with your feet about hip-distance apart.

2. Extend your arms down to your sides with your palms facing forward.

3. Slowly bend your elbows and bring your fingertips up to touch your shoulders, then release your arms back down to your starting point.

4. Repeat this movement three times.

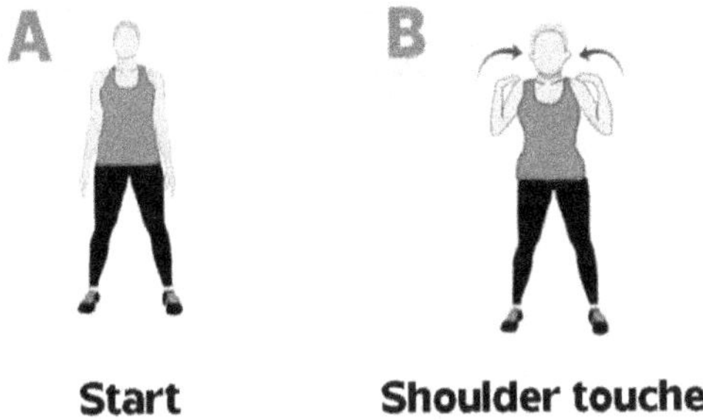

Start   **Shoulder touches**

Open and Close Hands

1. Begin standing tall with your arms out and down at your sides. Keep your palms facing forward.

2. Slowly open your fingers, stretching them as far as they can go without any discomfort, then close them tightly, making a fist.

3. Open and close your hands three times.

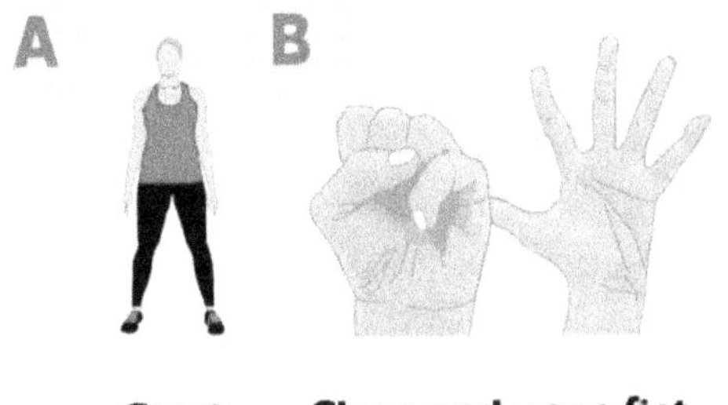

Start   **Close and open fist**

Leg Lift With Chair Support

1. Stand behind a chair with your feet hip-width apart and your hands holding onto the back of the chair for support.

2. Bending your right knee, lift your right leg back, then lower it. Now bend your left knee and lift your left leg back, and lower it.

3. Alternate doing this exercise between your right and left legs until you have done three repetitions.

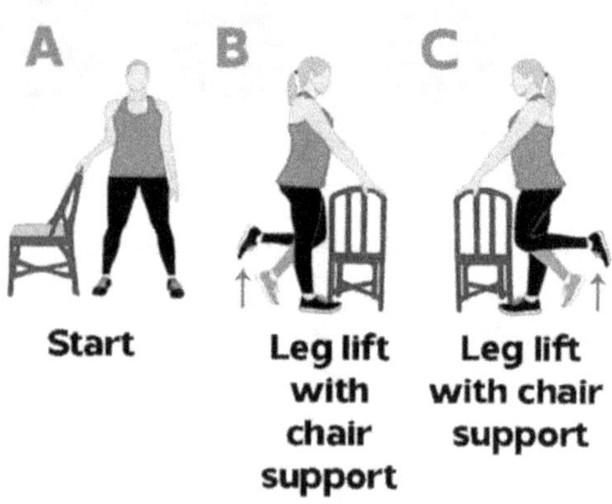

Crossed-Arm Rotation

1. Come to stand with your feet hip-distance apart and your toes pointing forward.

2. Cross your arms over your chest so your fingertips are touching opposite shoulders.

3. Keeping your lower body in place, slowly turn to your right, then return to center. Now turn to your left, and then back to center.

4. Repeat this movement three times on either side.

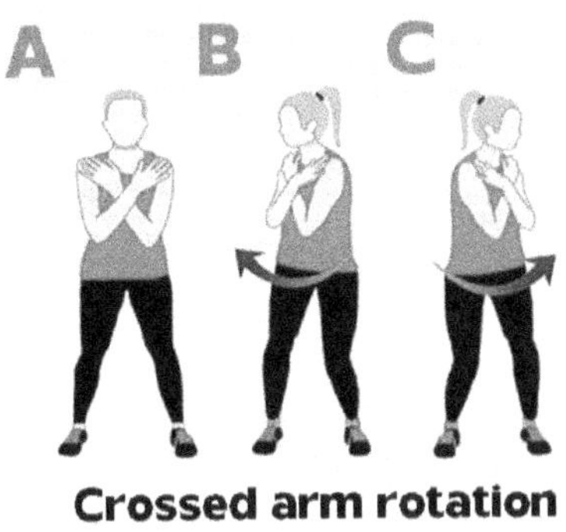

Crossed arm rotation

Calf Raises With Chair Support

1. Stand behind a chair and hold on to the chair back for support.

2. Slowly lift your heels off the floor as far as they can go then lower them back down with control.

3. Do this three times.

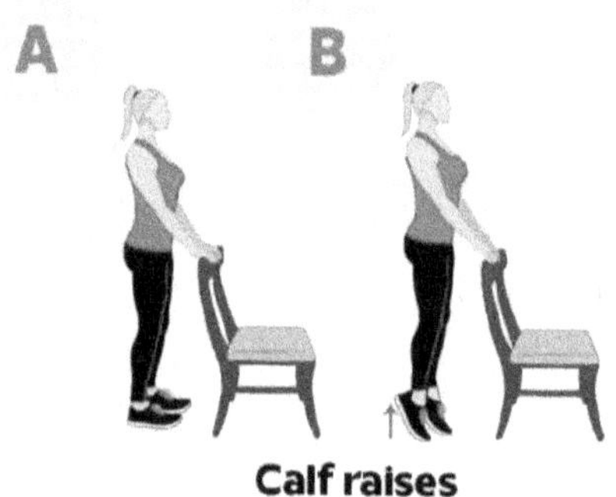

Calf raises

Seated Ankle Circles

1. Sit up tall in a chair with your knees bent at a 90-degree angle and your feet firmly planted on the floor.

2. Extend your right leg out in front of you, keeping your left leg as it is, for support.

3. Slowly begin to make circles with your right ankle in one direction for three counts, then reverse the circles and do three more.

4. Return your right leg to the starting position and extend your left leg in front of you. Repeat the ankle circles three times in both directions, then return to your start.

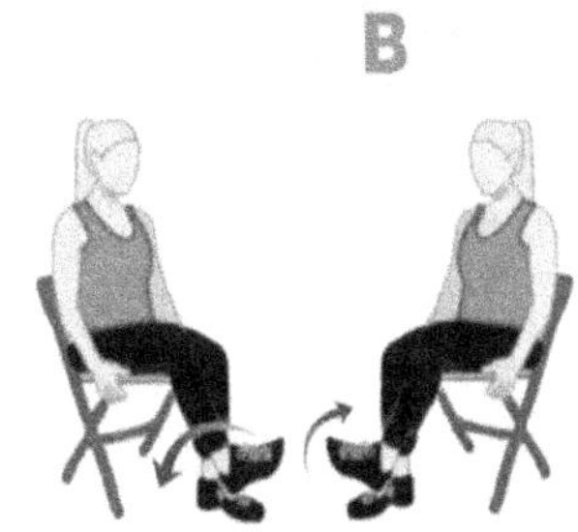

Seated ankle circles

Marching in Place

1. Stand with your feet hip-width apart and your toes pointing forward. Keep your arms down at your sides and your shoulders away from your ears.

2. Lift your right knee and lower it, then lift your left knee and lower it.

3. Swing opposite arms as you lift and lower your knees.

4. Continue marching on the spot for 30 seconds.

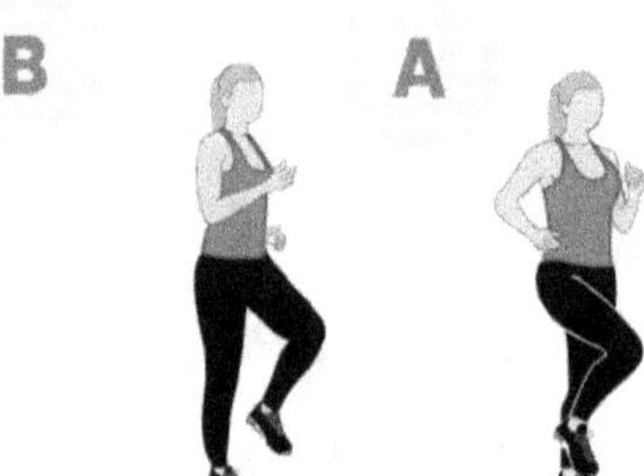

March in place

Chapter 4

The Importance of Hand, Neck, and Shoulder Exercises for Mobility

As older adults, we may begin to lose our ability to move easily or without discomfort. The recent global pandemic and the ensuing curtailment of freedom of movement, particularly for seniors, have taken a severe toll on our mobility. Not being able to go outdoors and exercise has led many older adults to complain about unsteadiness in performing their daily activities and tiring easily. Running errands or doing the grocery shopping have become exhausting tasks. All these issues may be attributed to reduced mobility which causes the hips, knees, and back to become stiff or tight. This, in turn, leads to muscle imbalances as well as reduced strength, stiffness, and pain in the muscles and joints.

It is especially important as we return to our daily lives that we begin to move again. Paying attention to exercises for increased mobility means that we will be able to get up from our bed or a chair, prepare a meal, have a shower, and get dressed—all without assistance. Improved mobility means self-sufficiency and independence.

The more we move, the better our muscle size, muscle length, and neural control become. This, in turn, means improved flexibility, which makes it easier for us to perform the basic tasks of caring for ourselves, like tying our laces, reaching for items on a shelf, or closing the trunk of the car.

When we know we can do chores by ourselves, it gives us confidence. Exercising to strengthen and stretch our muscles, therefore, leads to better mental health. Confidence in our mobility improves our cognitive function, boosting our memory, agility, and strategic thinking. It provides us with a sense of accomplishment and contribution.

As we age, our body's ability to absorb calcium is reduced and can result in osteoporosis (particularly for older women) and decreased bone mineralization (bone hardening). Exercise works for bones the same way it works for muscles—it strengthens them. Bone, like other living tissue, responds based on the pressure put on it. Therefore, the more regularly you exercise, the more bone you build and the denser it becomes. Moving and exercising daily can help fight osteoporosis, as well as promote bone mineralization. This means that if we do fall, there is less chance of broken bones or other injuries.

The older we get, the greater the chance of a fall or an injury. Improving our mobility, through stretching and strengthening, stabilizes the muscles that support us and helps us to perform our day-to-day endeavors. Furthermore, it can delay or reduce muscle loss.

Though this entire book focuses on strength training for seniors, the exercises in this chapter highlights routines for your legs, hands, neck, and shoulders. You can complete all of these routines together or you can build your routine choosing from different parts in order to get a whole body workout.

Seated Leg Exercises

If you have mobility concerns or balance issues, then seated exercises are a great alternative that can give you the same benefits. It still targets your lower body, but ensures your safety while doing the exercises.

Knee Extensions

1. Begin by sitting up tall in a chair with your arms relaxed at your sides. It would be better to use a chair without arms.

2. Slowly lift your right leg and straighten your right knee. Your right leg should be extended out in front of you. Only lift your leg as far as feels comfortable.

3. Hold here for three seconds, then release.

4. Switch legs and repeat this movement.

5. Do this exercise 15 times on each side.

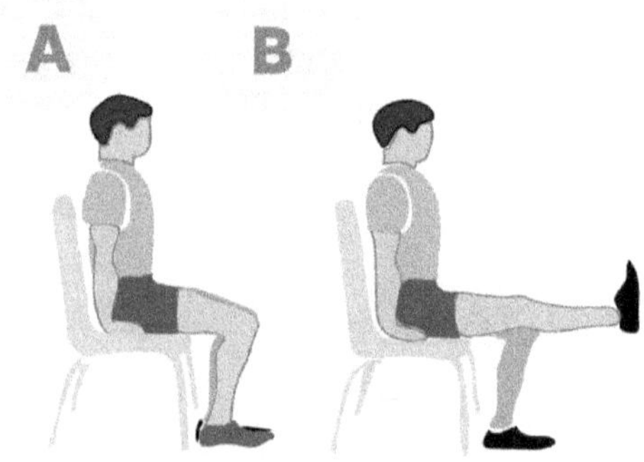

Knee extension

Pillow Squeeze

1. Sit in a chair with your arms relaxed at your sides and your back straight.

2. Your feet should be flat on the floor.

3. Place a pillow between your knees and squeeze the pillow by activating your thigh muscles.

4. Hold here for three seconds, then release.

5. Repeat this movement 12 times.

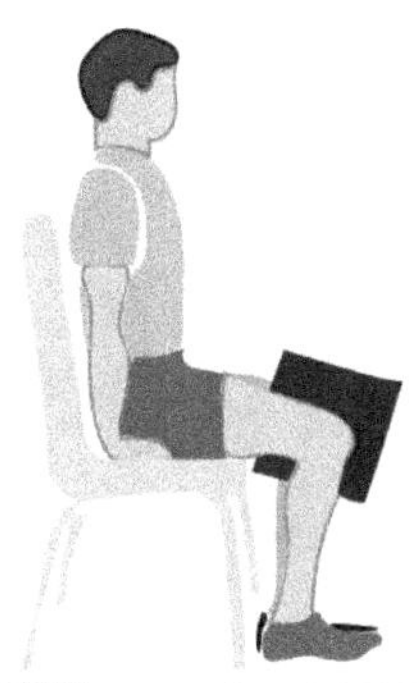

Pillow squeeze

Seated Clamshell

1. Begin by sitting up tall in a chair with your arms at your sides.

2. Keep your feet flat on the floor with your knees bent at a 90-degree angle.

3. Place your hands on the outsides of your knees so they act as resistance.

4. As you push your knees out away from each other, use your hands to push inward, creating resistance for your knees.

5. Hold this for three seconds, then relax.

6. Repeat this motion 12 times.

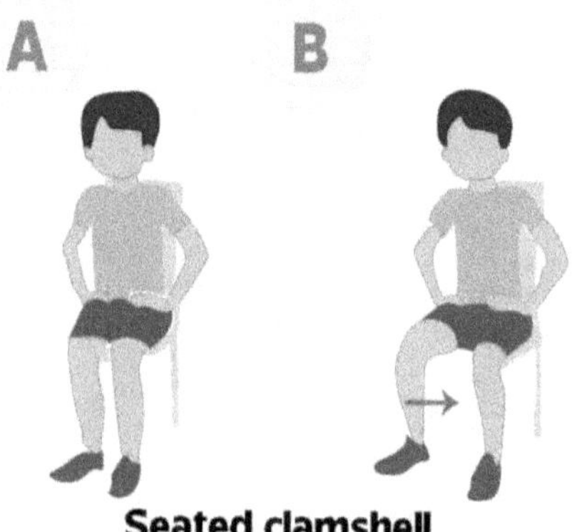

Seated clamshell

Straight Knee Ankle Pumps

1. Begin by sitting tall in a chair with your arms at your sides.

2. Extend both legs out in front of you with your heels touching the floor and your toes pointing toward the ceiling.

3. Flex your toes and hold for three seconds, then point your toes and hold for three seconds.

4. Repeat this exercise ten times in each direction.

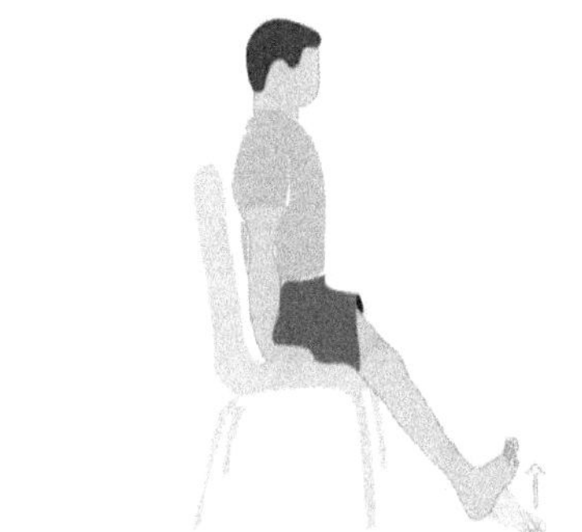

Straight knee ankle pumps

Seated Marching

1. Sit up tall in your chair with your arms relaxed at your side.

2. Place your feet flat on the floor with your knees hip-width apart.

3. Begin to march, lifting one leg up then the other, as high as you can go. If you can, swing the opposite arms as you march in your seat.

4. Complete at least 20 full marches, or march for at least 30 seconds.

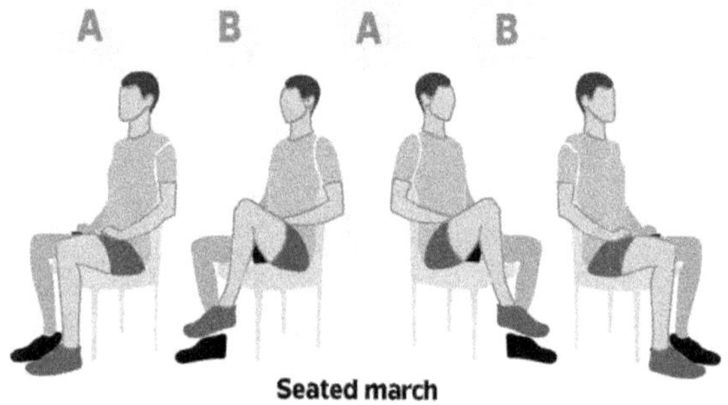

Seated march

Hand and Finger Stretches

It may not seem important at first, but stretching and strengthening your hands and fingers are crucial if you want to continue performing your daily activities. The exercises here will ensure you can perform fine motor skills like picking things up and even holding your fork.

Make a Fist

1. Make a fist with your right hand, wrapping your thumb across your finger.

2. Hold this fist for 30 seconds, then release, spreading your fingers wide.

3. Do this movement four times with your right hand, then switch and repeat with your left hand.

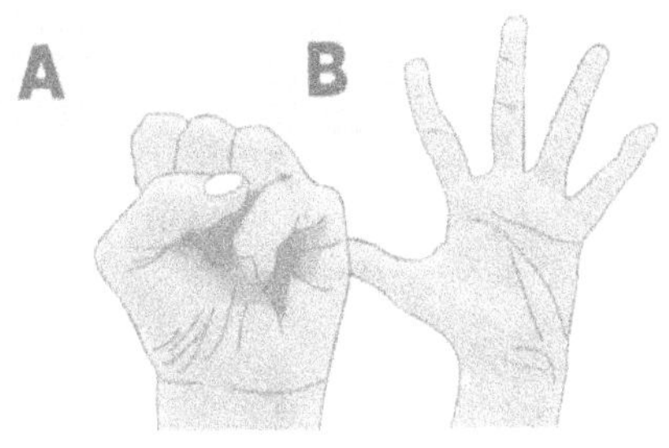

Make a fist

Finger Stretches

1. Sit at a table and place your right hand on the table with your palm facing down.

2. Straighten your fingers as much as you can without forcing or feeling any pain or discomfort.

3. Hold your hand open here for 30 seconds, then relax your fingers.

4. Perform this stretch four times with your right hand, and then repeat with your left hand.

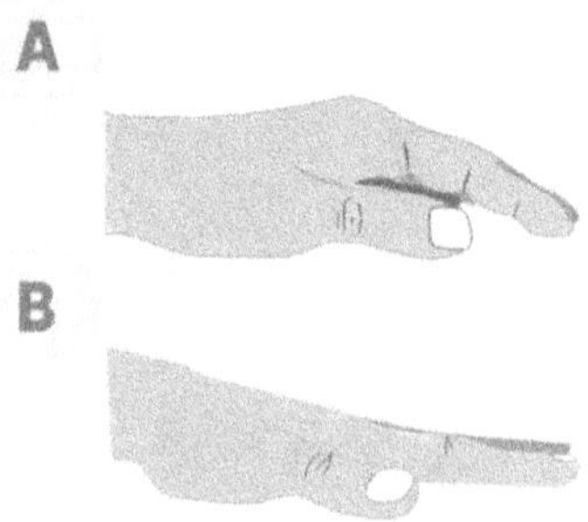

Finger stretches

Claw Stretch

1. Sit comfortably and hold your right hand out in front of you with the palm facing in.

2. Bend your fingers down and in, as you reach your fingertips to the base of your finger joints. Your hand should look a bit like a claw.

3. Hold this claw-shape for 30 seconds, then release your fingers.

4. Do this four times with your right hand, then repeat with your left hand.

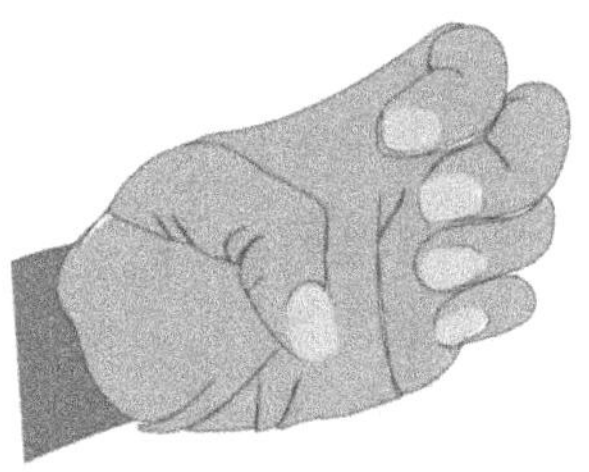

Claw stretch

Grip Strengthening

1. Hold a small, soft ball in your right hand.

2. Now squeeze it as hard as you can. Hold here for a few seconds, then release.

3. Perform this movement ten times with each hand.

4. Try to do this exercise two to three times a week, giving yourself 48 hours between sessions.

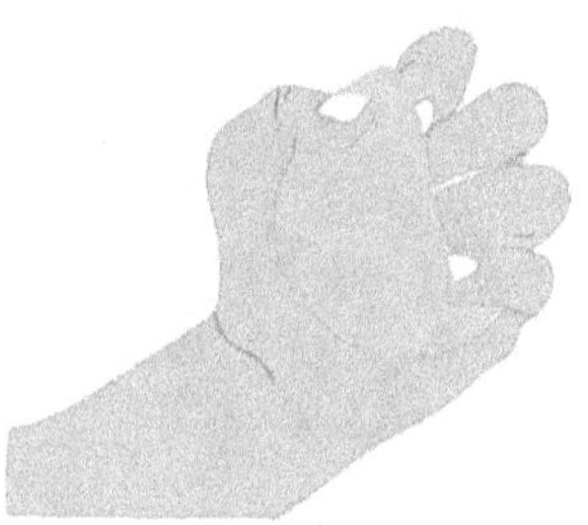

Grip strengthening

Pinch Strengthening

1. Hold a small, soft ball in your right hand and pinch it between your thumb and fingers.

2. Hold here for 30 seconds, then relax your grip.

3. Repeat this exercise ten times with each hand.

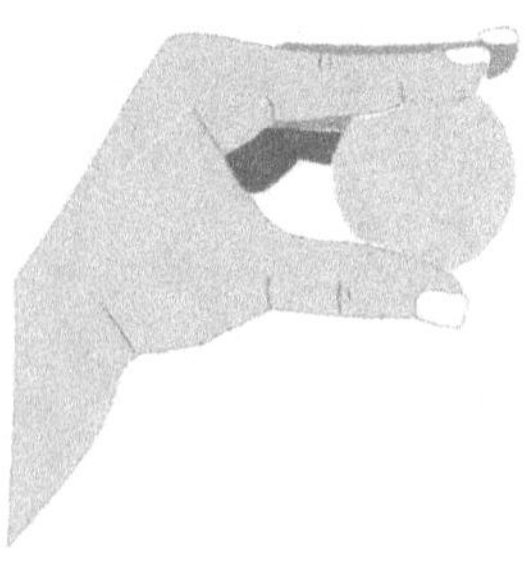

Pinch strengthening

Finger Lifts

1. Sitting at a table, place your right hand on the table with your palm facing down.

2. Slowly lift and lower one finger at a time, keeping your palm and other fingers on the table until you've done all your fingers.

3. Do this 8 to 12 times with one hand, then repeat with the other hand.

4. You can also try lifting and lowering all your fingers on your hand and your thumb at once.

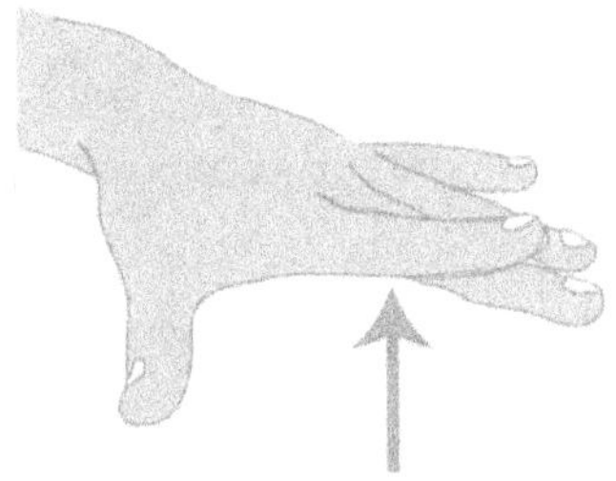

Finger lifts

Thumb Extensions

1. Sit comfortably at a table.

2. Wrap an elastic band around your right hand near the base of your finger joints, so that your fingers are all together.

3. Slowly move your thumb away from your fingers as far as you can.

4. Hold here for 30 seconds, then release. Do this 8 to 12 times.

5. Repeat with your left hand.

6. This exercise can be done two to three times per week, with a 48-hour rest time between sessions.

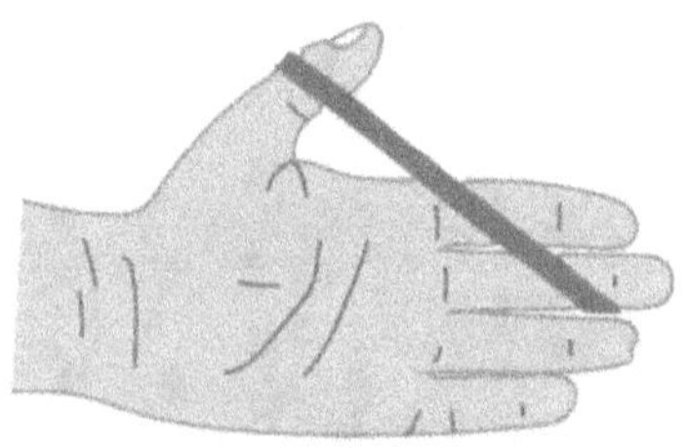

Thumb extension

Thumb Flex

1. Put your right hand out in front of you with your palm facing up.

2. Move your thumb as far away from your fingers as you can. Now bend your thumb across your palm and try to touch the base of your little finger.

3. Hold here for 30 seconds, then release.

4. Do this four times with each hand.

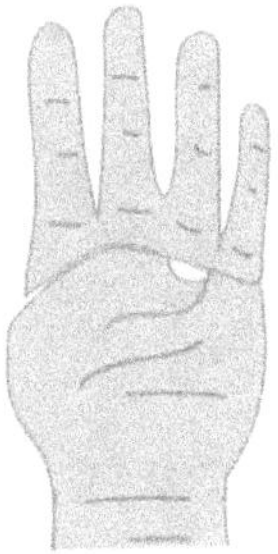

Thumb flex

Thumb Touch

1. Hold your right hand up with your palm facing forward and your wrist straight.

2. Touch your right thumb to each of your fingertips (one at a time), forming an 'o' shape. Pause for 30 seconds on each finger, then move on to the next.

3. Repeat this exercise four times on each hand.

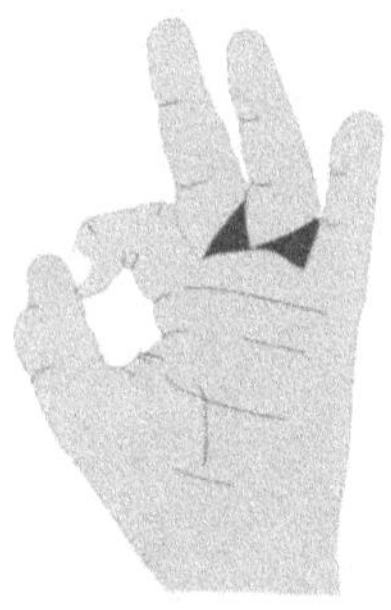

Thumb touch

Thumb Stretches

1. Hold your right hand out in front of you with your palm facing toward you.

2. Slowly bend your thumb down to the base of your index finger.

3. Hold here for 30 seconds then release. Do it four more times.

4. Still holding your right hand out in front of you, stretch your right thumb across your palm, only using your lower thumb joint.

5. Hold for 30 seconds, then release. Repeat four more times.

6. Switch to your left hand and complete the same movements.

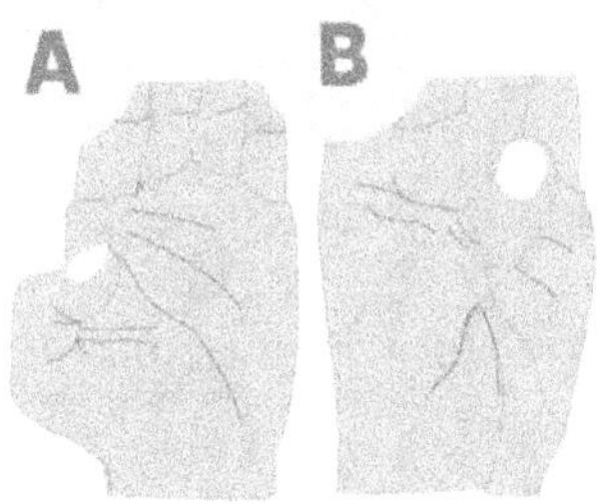

Thumb stretch

Neck Exercises

We may take our neck for granted, but it performs the important task of holding our head up. We may even spend large swathes of time with our heads bent forward and our shoulders hunched, creating additional tension in our necks. Stretching our neck can reduce this tension and stiffness, and improve its overall function, as well as our quality of life.

Neck Retraction

1. Sit with your back straight in a comfortable chair.

2. Place two fingers on your chin.

3. Gently apply pressure to your chin with your fingers so that you push your head straight

back. You should feel a stretch at the back of your neck.

4. Hold here for four seconds, then release.

5. Perform this movement ten times.

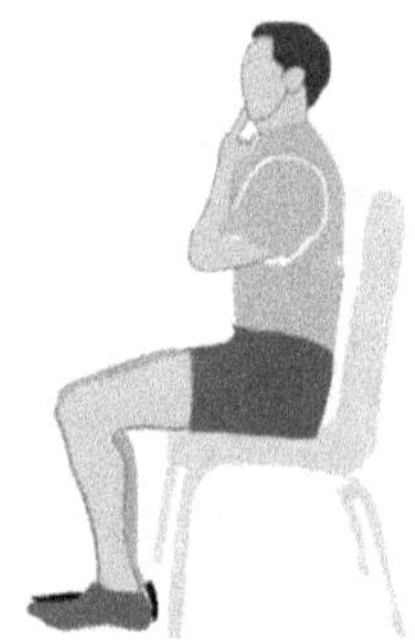

Neck retraction

Seated Cervical Rotation

1. Sit up tall in a chair and place the middle and index fingers of your right hand on your right chin.

2. Slowly push your chin towards your left shoulder.

3. Hold here for ten seconds, then release back to your starting position.

4. Repeat this ten more times, then switch to your left side.

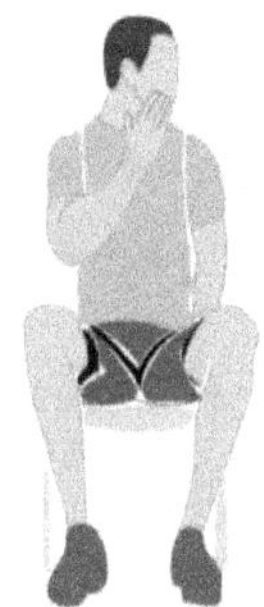

Seated cervical rotation

Shoulder Squeeze

1. Stand with your feet hip-width apart and your arms relaxed down at your sides.

2. Squeeze your shoulder blades together so that your chest opens up.

3. Hold here for ten seconds, then relax your shoulders.

4. Repeat this motion ten times.

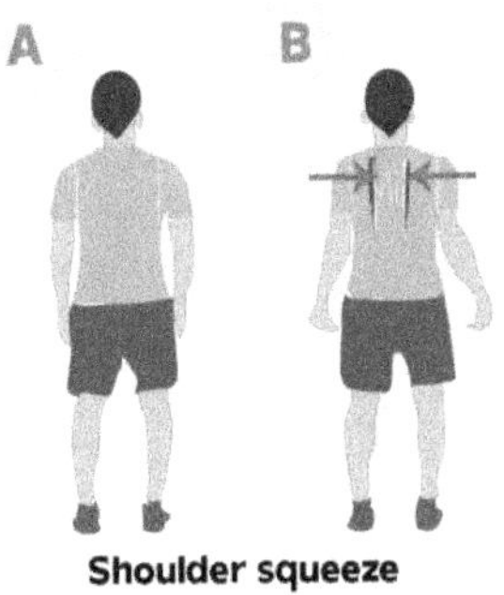

Shoulder squeeze

Shoulder Rolls

1. Begin by standing with your feet hip-distance apart and your arms down at your sides.

2. Slowly make circles with your shoulders in a clockwise direction.

3. After completing ten repetitions in this direction, reverse your circles and do ten more in a counterclockwise direction.

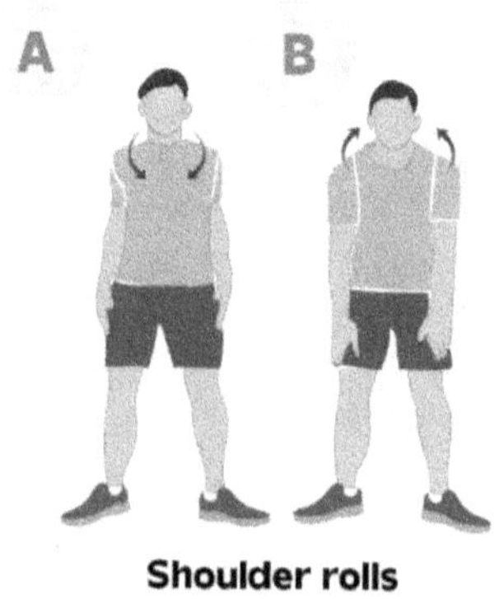

Shoulder rolls

Shoulder Exercises

We may not be able to stop the aging process, but we can certainly delay its effects. Strengthening our shoulder muscles means that we can slow or reverse loss of muscle mass in our arms and shoulders. It makes eating, gardening, playing with our grandkids, and generally moving easier and pain-free.

Diagonal Outward Shoulder Lift

1. Begin in a standing position with your feet hip-distance apart.

2. Place a two-pound weight in your right hand and bring it near to your left hip, keeping your palm facing inward. Your left arm can relax at your side.

3. Slowly extend your arm up and across your body over to your right side, then lower it back to your starting position.

4. Repeat this movement ten times, then switch and do it with your left arm.

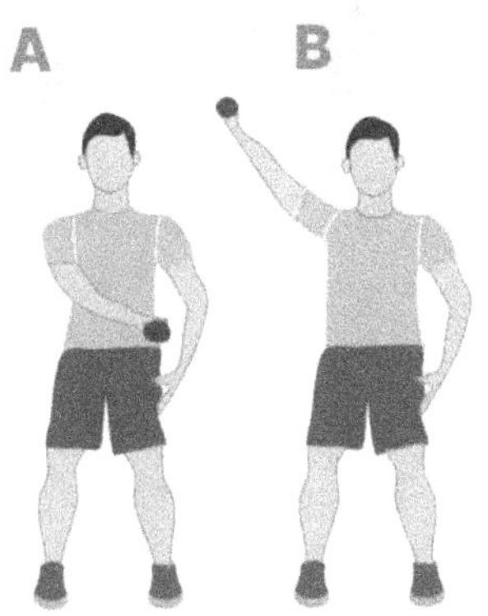

Diagonal outward shoulder lift

Bicep Curls

1. Stand with your feet hip-width apart and your feet firmly pressing into the floor.

2. Hold a two-pound weight in your right hand and lower your arms to your sides with your palms facing inward.

3. Keep your shoulders down and your chest open.

4. As you breathe out, slowly bend your right elbow and bring the weight up toward your right shoulder, turning your palm toward your chest.

5. Gently lower your arm back down to your starting position as you breathe in.

6. Complete ten repetitions on your right side, then switch the weight over to your left and repeat the movement.

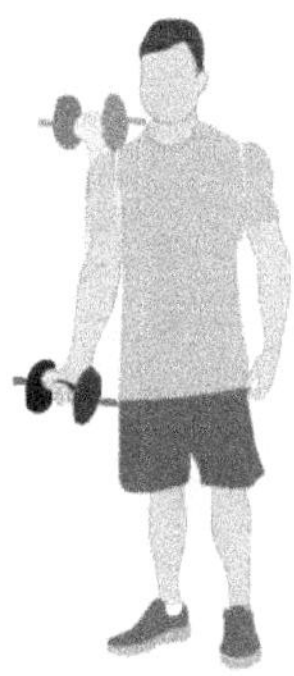

Bicep curl

Upright Row

1. Stand with your feet hip-distance apart and your toes facing forward.

2. Hold weights in both your hands and bring your hands in front of your hips.

3. Breathe out and slowly lift the weights as if you are sliding them up the front of your body until they are just under your chin. Your elbows should be pointing out to either side.

4. Gently lower them back down as you breathe in.

5. Repeat this motion ten times.

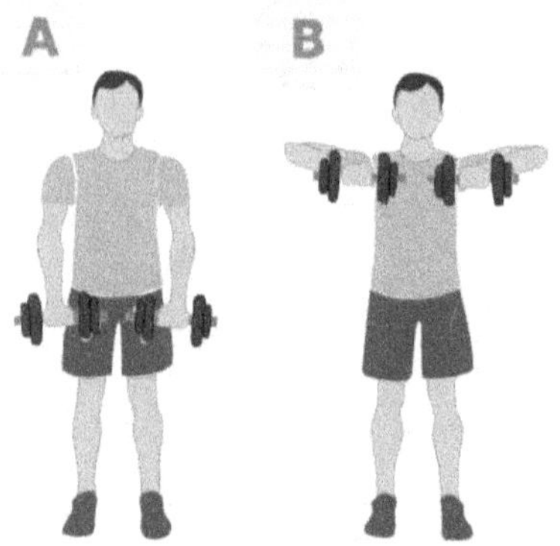

Upright row

Diagonal Inward Shoulder Lift

1. Come to stand with your feet hip-width apart.

2. Place a weight in your right hand and hold it down at your side with your palm facing forward.

3. Slowly lift your arm up and across your body toward your left shoulder, bending your elbow and turning your palm in.

4. Lower your right arm back to your starting position.

5. Perform this lift ten times, then switch the weight to your left hand and repeat.

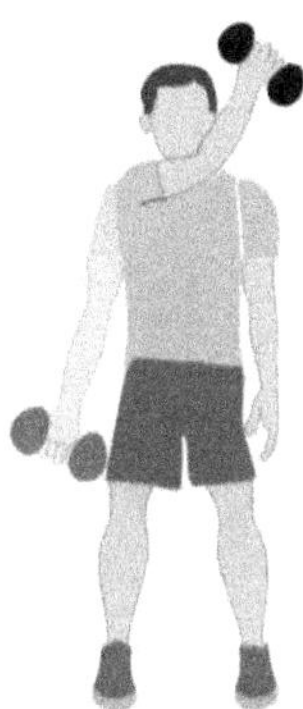

Diagonal inward shoulder lift

Bent Over Row

1. Stand in front of a chair and hold onto the chair back with your left hand.

2. Hold the weight in your right hand at your side with your palm facing in and lean over the chair, using your left hand to support you.

3. Slowly lift your right arm back until your elbow is the same height as your shoulder and the weight is near your chest as you exhale. Then, release back to the start as you inhale.

4. Do this ten times, then switch to the left side and repeat.

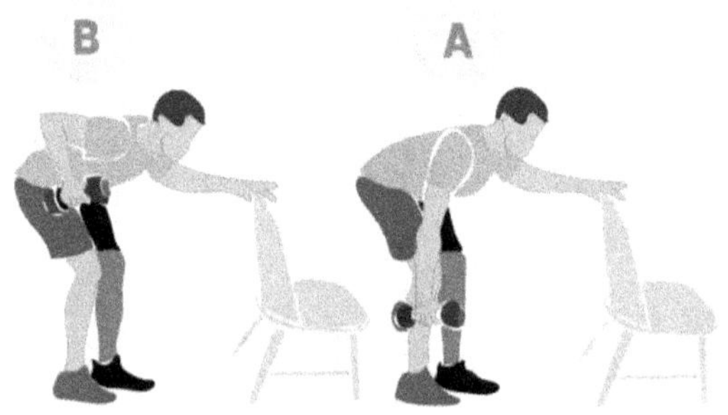

Bent over row

Overhead Elbow Extension

1. Stand with your legs hip-width apart and your feet firmly pressed into the floor.

2. Hold the weight in your right hand and lift your arm until the weight is near your right shoulder and your elbow is pointing forward. Keep your palm facing inward.

3. On an exhale, slowly straighten your arm to lift the weight over your head. You can hold your right elbow with your left hand for support.

4. Inhale and gently lower your weight back down to your starting position.

5. Repeat this ten times, then switch to the other side.

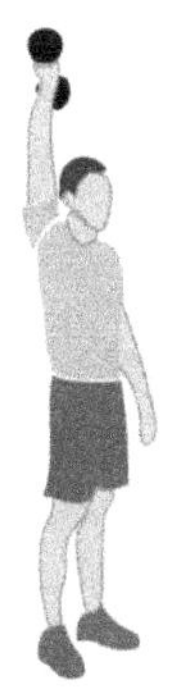

Overhead elbow extension

Shoulder Rolls

1. Begin by standing with your feet hip-distance apart and hold weights in each hand, lowering your arms along your sides.

2. Lift your shoulders up toward your ears as you inhale, then roll them back and down as you exhale.

3. Repeat this shoulder roll 20 times.

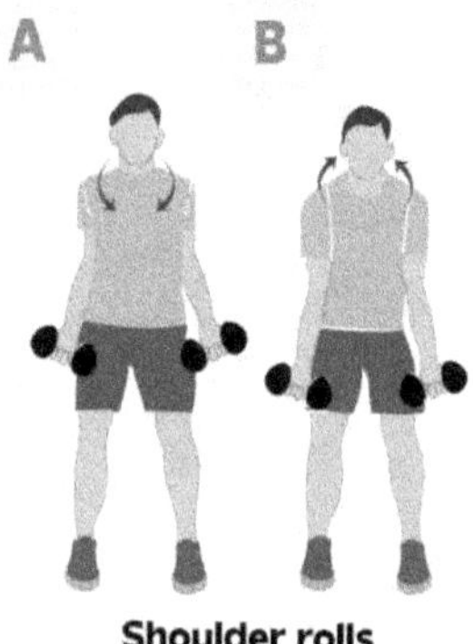

Shoulder rolls

Triceps Kickback

1. Stand behind a chair and lean over it, placing your left hand on the back of the chair to support you. Hold a two-pound weight in your right hand.

2. Bend your right elbow so that your upper arm is tucked in close to your side and your lower arm is at a right angle. Keep your palm facing inward.

3. Straighten your elbow, extending your right arm behind you as far as feels comfortable on an exhale, then inhale as you return to your starting position.

4. Do this ten times with your right arm, then switch and repeat on your left side.

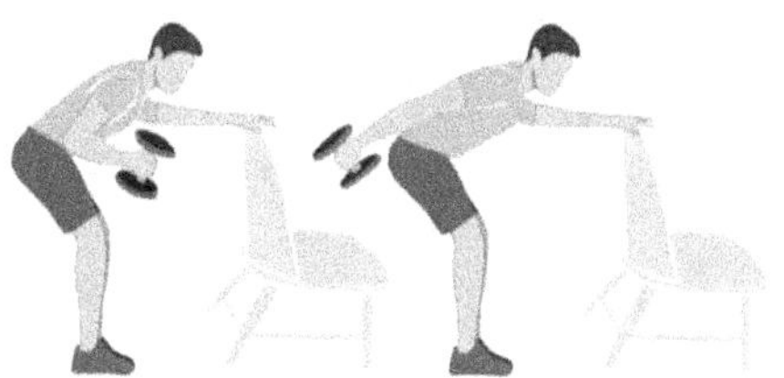

Triceps kickback

Overhead Press

1. Stand with your feet shoulder-distance apart and your toes pointing forward.

2. Hold a two-pound weight in each hand at chest level. with your palms facing forward.

3. As you exhale, slowly lift both arms up over your head at the same time, then inhale and lower back down to your starting point.

4. Repeat this exercise ten times.

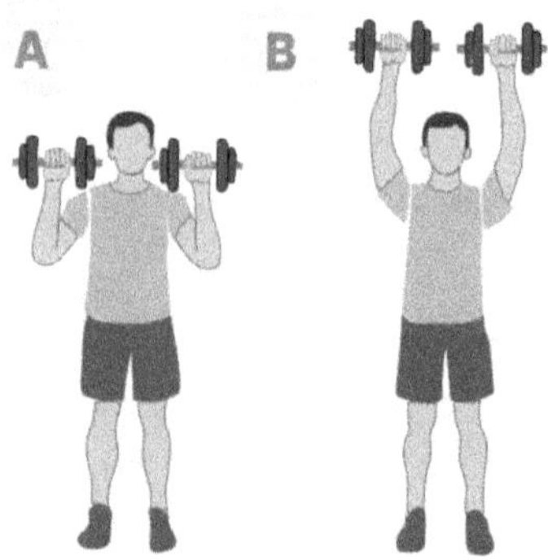

Overhead press

Shoulder Press Lying Down

1. Lie on the floor on your back with your legs extended out. Make sure to keep your head, back, and butt firmly pressing into the floor.

2. Hold a two-pound weight in each hand and bend your elbows so they are at 90-degree angles and your palms are facing inward.

3. Exhale and slowly lift both arms toward the ceiling with your elbows pointing out.

4. Gently lower back down to your starting position as you inhale.

5. Perform this exercise ten times.

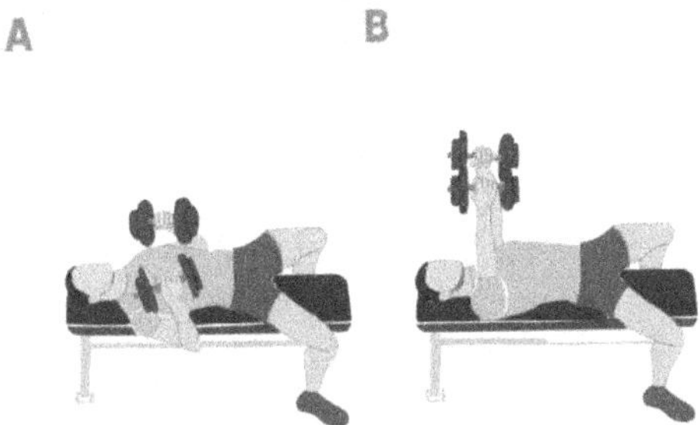

Shouldre press lying down

Side Shoulder Raise

1. Stand with your feet hip-width apart.

2. Hold a two-pound weight in your right arm and lower your arm down your side with your palm facing forward.

3. Slowly lift your right arm out to the side and over your head on an exhale, then lower it back down as you inhale.

4. Complete ten repetitions on your right side, then switch to your left.

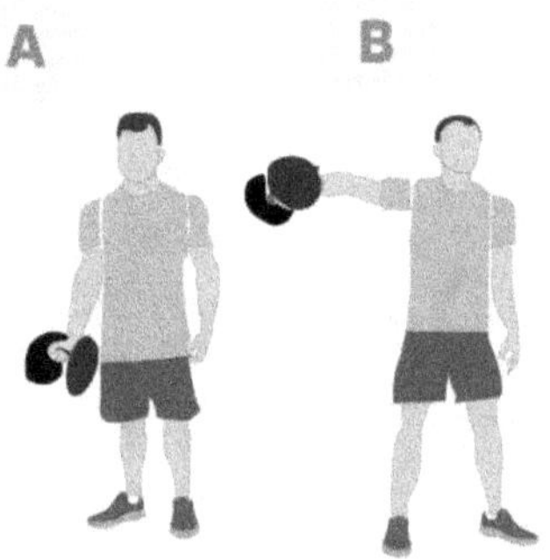

Side shoulder raise

Elbow Side Extensions

1. Begin by standing with your legs shoulder-distance apart and your feet flat on the floor.

2. Hold a weight in each hand and bring the weights to your chest with your palms facing inward. Your elbows should be pointing out to the sides.

3. Exhale and slowly straighten both arms out to the sides at the same time, then return to center as you inhale.

4. Repeat this ten times.

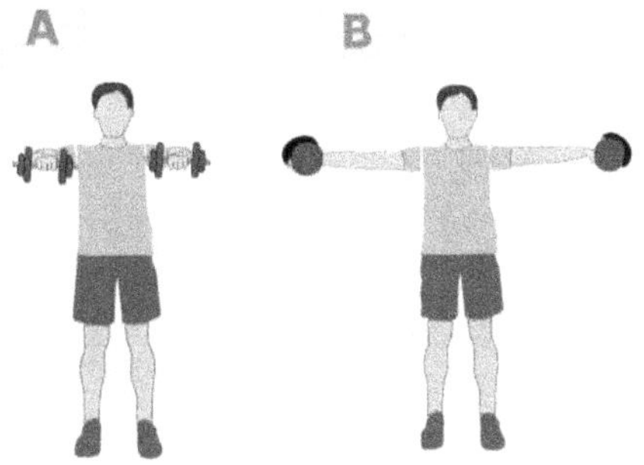

Elbow side extension

Chapter 5:

The Tangible Benefits of

Upper and Lower Body

Exercises

We all know that regular exercise is important, but it becomes even more critical as we get older. Have you ever tried to open a jar of olives? Then you know how important strong muscles are. Weak muscles mean that we are more susceptible to pain and injury. In fact, according to the American Chiropractic Association, back pain is the second most cited reason for visiting the doctor (Healthline, 2014). In most instances, the back pain is a mechanical issue as opposed to an infection, illness, or injury. In some cases, it can be a result of arthritis, extra weight, poor posture, or stress.

When you have back pain or any other kind of pain, daily tasks and activities become increasingly difficult, which can make us more dependent on others for help. A lack of activity can cause our chest muscles to tighten, our back muscles to loosen, and our shoulders to hunch forward. It can also cause imbalances in our muscles, which can restrict our movements. By exercising and moving regularly, we can keep our muscles strong and our spine limber.

Daily exercise can improve our heart health by increasing the level of oxygen flowing to our cells and available for our use. It can reduce or even repair the damage to our arteries caused by high blood pressure, high blood sugar, and cholesterol. All of this means that we can lower our risk of heart disease or heart attack.

For most of us as we age, our continued independence is of utmost importance. Having a strong, functioning upper and lower body means that we can carry our own groceries, do our own gardening, delay the onset of illness, and, in general, be self-sufficient. Daily movement ensures that we can reduce the loss of muscle mass usually associated with aging, and increase our flexibility, which means fewer aches and pains overall.

When you haven't been active in a while, or if you experience pain, doing floor exercises can be difficult and uncomfortable. The exercises in this section can be performed standing or seated to help you get moving. Standing exercises can also strengthen your glutes, which work intimately with your core muscles. You can perform these exercises in the order they appear, or you can switch it up to suit your needs or your mood. These exercises have been chosen to get you moving toward your independence.

Seated Stretches for Back Pain

A great way to delay or prevent back pain is to ensure that our postural muscles remain strong and our spine remains supple. This seated routine for your back targets the muscles along your spine, as well as other areas of your back, helping you to manage and alleviate any discomfort you may be experiencing.

Neck and Chest Stretch

1. Begin by sitting up straight on an armless chair. Make sure that your feet are flat on the floor.

2. Bring your hands to the back of your head and interlace your fingers, leaving your thumbs out along the sides of your neck. Your elbows should be pointing out to the side.

3. Relax your head back into your hands, and lift your chin up toward the ceiling.

4. As you inhale, gently bend to your left so that your left elbow is tipping toward the ground and your right elbow is lifting up to the ceiling. You should feel a gentle stretch along the side of the neck. It should not feel painful in any way.

5. Take two breaths in this position, then slowly lift yourself back up to your starting position.

6. Repeat these movements on your right side.

7. Alternate your movements on each side as you complete this move three times on each side.

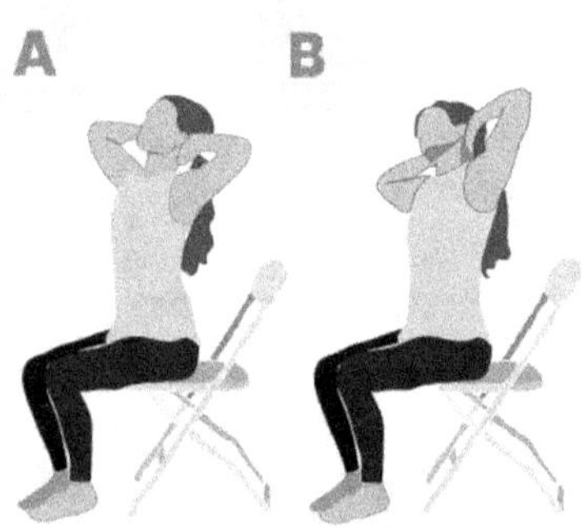

Neck and chest stretch

Seated Backbend

1. Sit up tall in an armless chair with your feet firmly pressing into the floor. Don't sit all the way back in the chair.

2. Place your palms on your lower back with your fingers facing down and your thumbs around your hips.

3. As you inhale, press your palms into your lower back.

4. On your exhale, slowly arch your spine by raising your chin up and lifting your face to the ceiling. Try not to let your head drop back too much. You should have the sensation of going up and over a ball.

5. Hold your backbend for five deep breaths.

6. Gently release and return to your seated position.

7. Repeat this bend three to five times.

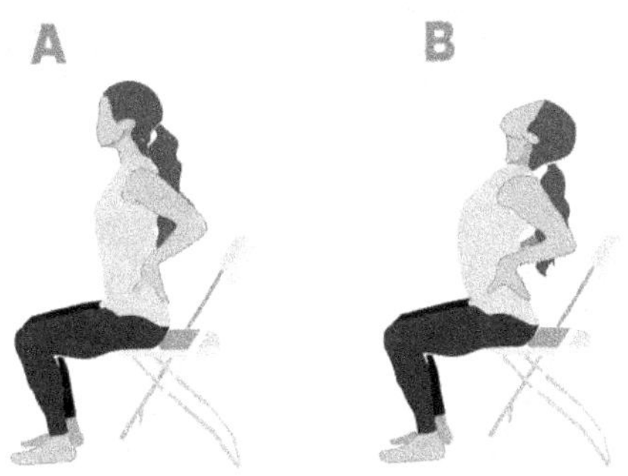

Seated backbend

Shoulder and Chest Stretch

1. Sit up straight in a chair with your feet flat on the floor.

2. Inhale, and on your exhale, reach behind you and link your fingers together. If linking your

fingers is difficult, you can hold on to your wrists or elbows.

3. On your next inhale, sit up taller and roll your shoulders back, bringing your shoulder blades down along your back.

4. Exhale and straighten your arms, keeping your fingers interlaced. If you are holding your elbows, gently pull in opposite directions to open up your upper back and chest.

5. Hold here for three breaths, then slowly release.

6. Repeat these motions three more times.

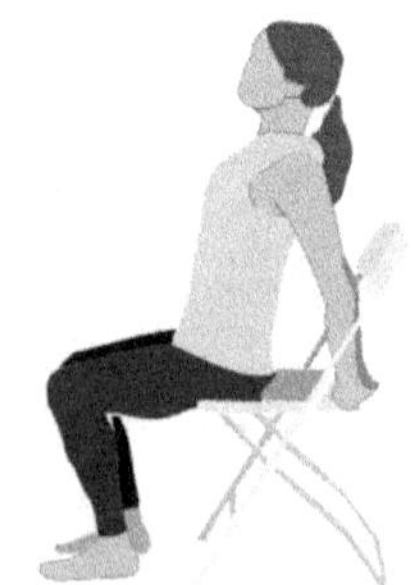

Shoulder and chest stretch

Seated Cat-Cow

1. Begin by sitting on an armless chair with your feet firmly pressed into the floor and your knees

hip-width apart. Your knees should be at a 90-degree angle with your ankles directly under your knees.

2. Rest your hands, palms down, on your knees, with your fingers facing in toward each other. The heels of your hands should be on the outside of your legs.

3. Inhale deeply and begin to lift your chin up toward the ceiling, arching your back and dropping your shoulders away from your ears.

4. As you exhale, drop your chin toward your chest, roll your shoulders forward, and round your back, pushing your palms into your knees.

5. Repeat these movements slowly, following your breath, three to five times.

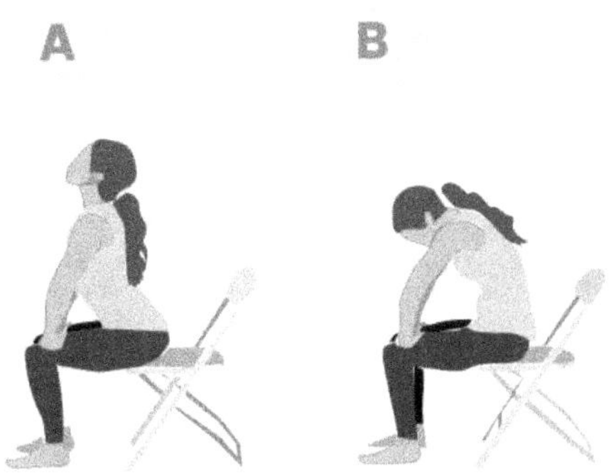

Seated cat-cow

Gentle Seated Twist

1. Start by sitting up tall in a chair with your feet
    flat on the floor and your knees hip-width apart.
    Come forward a bit in your chair, so that you
    have some room behind you, but not so far that
    you feel as if you may tip over.

2. Inhale and lift your arms up over your head.
    Keep your shoulders down, away from your
    ears, and keep your spine straight and tall.

3. Exhale slowly as you turn to your right. Put
    your left hand on the outside of your right knee
    and your right hand on the back of the chair (or
    wherever feels most comfortable). You should
    feel a gentle twist. Try not to crank your body
    as you turn.

4. Inhale again in the twist and try to sit up taller,
    maybe even deepening the twist as you exhale.

5. Take three to five deep breaths in your twist
    and then slowly return to your starting position.

6. Repeat the twist on your left side, placing your
    right hand on the outside of your left knee and
    your left hand on the back of the chair.

7. Alternate doing this twist three times on each
    side.

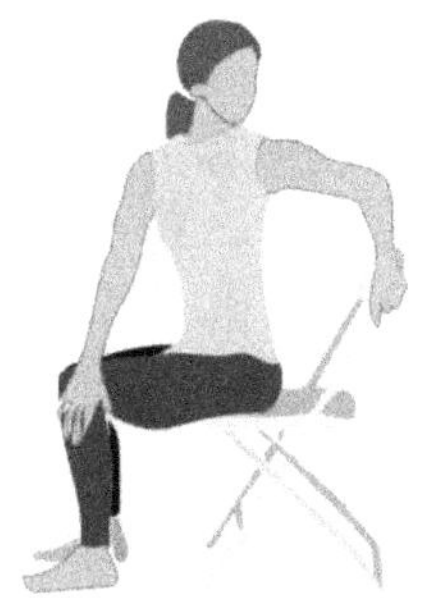

Gentle seated twist

Standing Core Exercises for Upper Back

In order to prevent us from placing too much stress on our back muscles, we need to have a strong core. Moreover, if you're suffering from back pain, lying on the floor to do core work is difficult or impossible. This standing core routine strengthens your core as well as the muscles of your glutes, both of which work collaboratively with your back muscles in order to support you and enable you to perform your daily tasks.

Reverse Dumbbell Woodchops

1. Stand with your feet hip-width apart and hold the dumbbell with both hands down in front of you.

2. Hinging at your hips and bending your knees, slightly rotate your body to the right and lower the dumbbell toward your right leg.

3. Keeping your core active, raise your arms diagonally so that the dumbbell is over your head on your left, and at the same time, rotate your left foot inward.

4. Lower to your starting position.

5. Repeat this exercise eight times on your right side, then switch to your left.

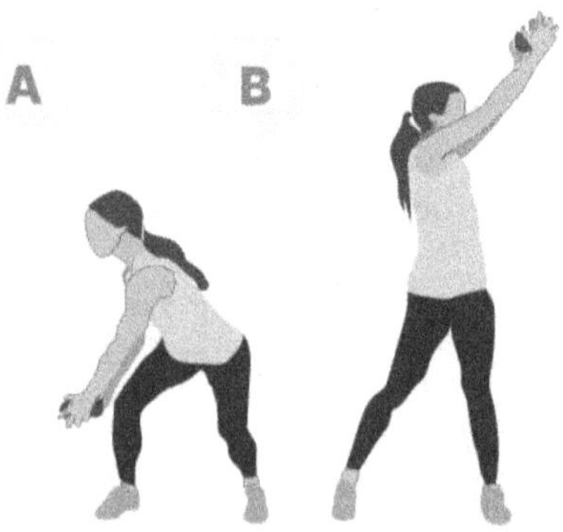

Reverse dumbell woodchops

Side-to-Side Rotations

1. Stand with your feet hip-width apart and hold a two-pound weight with both hands.

2. Engaging your core muscles, then lift your arms up and out in front of you.

3. Slowly move your arms from left to right, rotating your right foot in when your arms move to the left, and your left foot in when your arms move to the right.

4. Repeat this movement eight times for two sets.

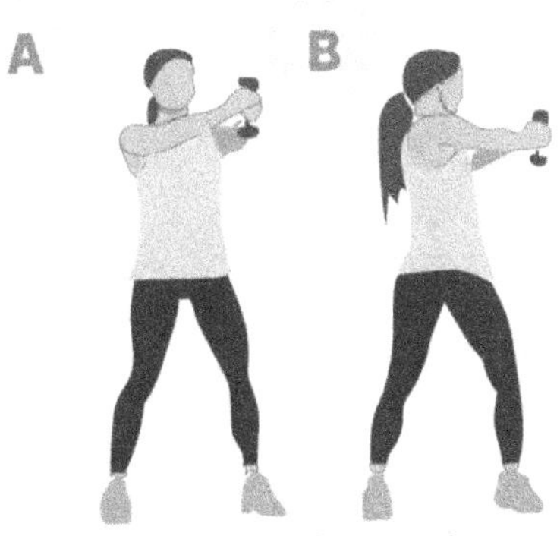

Side to side rotations

Figure 8

1. Begin with your feet hip-distance apart and hold a two-pound dumbbell with both hands.

2. Lift your arms up so that the dumbbell is at chest-level, then extend your arms out so that the weight is away from you.

3. Slowly begin to trace a figure 8 with the dumbbell. Try to keep your body stable as you do this.

4. Continue this exercise for one minute.

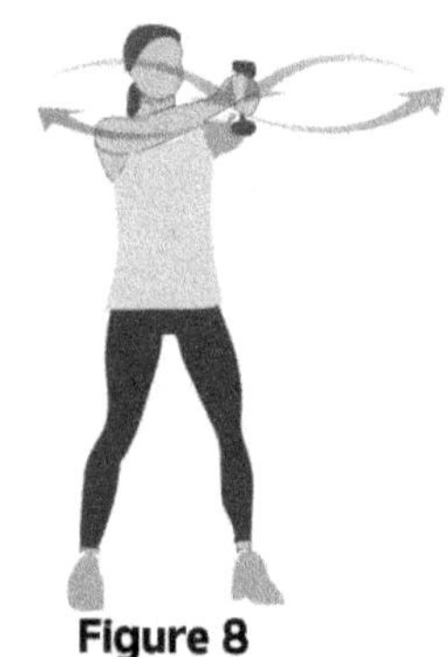

Figure 8

Knee to Elbow

1. Begin with your feet slightly wider than hip-distance apart. Interlace your fingers behind your head, so that your elbows are pointing out to the sides.

2. Stand up tall and engage the muscles of your core.

3. Lift your right knee up and out to the side as you tilt your right elbow down to meet your right knee, then return to your starting position.

4. Do this eight times on your right side, then switch to your left side.

5. Complete two sets of this exercise.

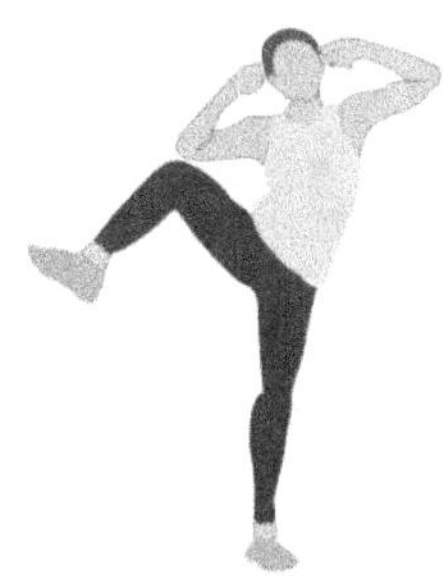

Knee to elbow

Leg Lifts

1. Come to stand with your feet together and your arms crossed over your chest.

2. Shift your weight to your left leg as you lift your right leg out to the side at a 45 degree angle. Make sure you are not collapsing into your left hip as you lift your right leg.

3. Gently lower your leg back down.

4. Repeat this eight times with your right leg, then switch to your left.

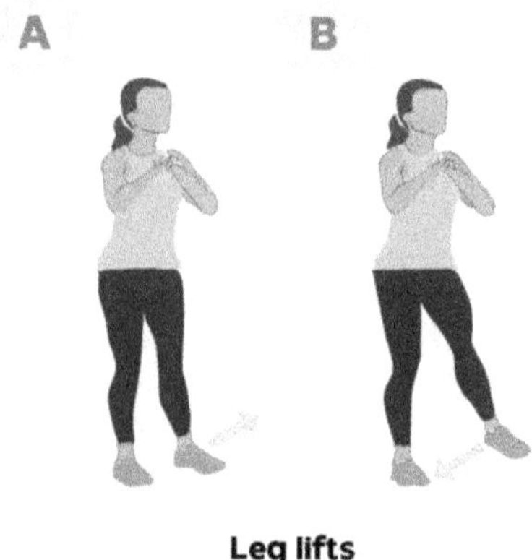

Leg lifts

Backward Lunge to Side Rotation

1. Begin by standing with your feet hip-width apart and your toes facing forward. Cross your arms in front of you, keeping your elbows lifted away from your body.

2. Step back into a lunge with your right foot.

3. Now rotate your upper body to the left. Keep your balance by activating the muscles of your core and your glutes.

4. Return your upper body to its starting position and bring your right foot back up to standing.

5. Repeat these movements with your left leg.

6. Complete this exercise eight times on each side.

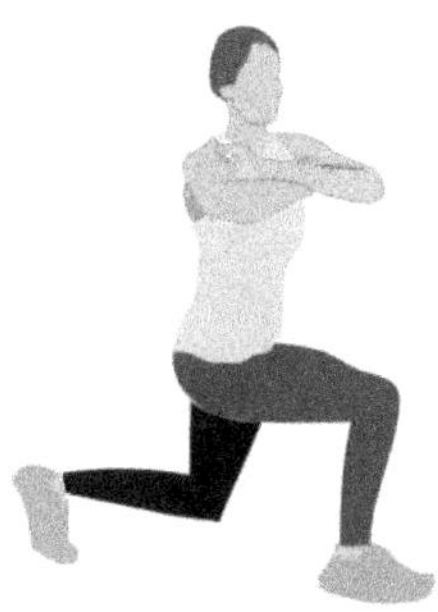

Backwards lunge to side rotation

Seated Lower Back Exercises

This workout focuses on the muscles of your lower back. Strong muscles in your lower back help to reduce your chances of back pain and makes it easier to perform tasks like lifting, sitting, and getting up.

Shoulder Rolls

1. Sit slightly forward in an armless chair with your feet flat on the floor.

2. Let your hands rest comfortably on your thighs.

3. Roll your shoulders up, back, down, and around.

4. Repeat rolling your shoulders back ten times, then reverse the movement and roll your shoulders forward ten times.

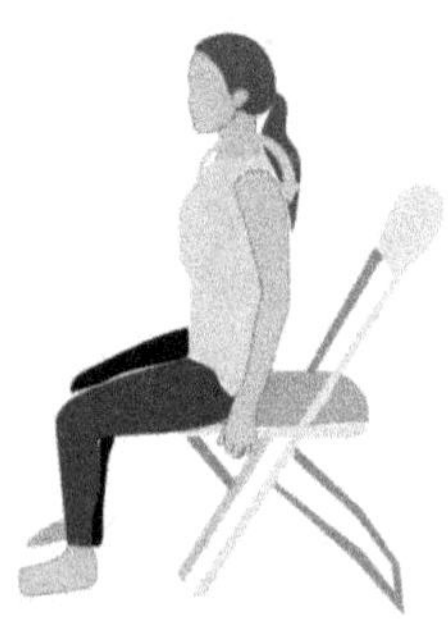

Shoulder rolls

Seated Toe Touch

1. Begin by sitting slightly forward in your chair with your feet firmly pressed into the floor. Keep your back straight.

2. Inhale and lift your arms up over your head (or as far as feels comfortable).

3. As you exhale, lean forward, lowering your arms toward your toes. You don't have to touch your toes; just go as far as feels good for you.

4. Inhale and lift back up to your starting position.

5. Repeat this movement ten times.

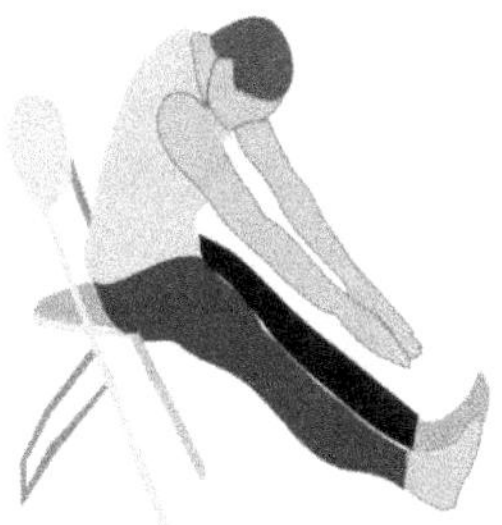

Seated toe touch

Side Stretch

1. Sit forward on your chair with your knees hip-width apart and your feet flat on the floor.

2. Place your hands behind your head with your elbows pointing out to the sides like triangles.

3. Inhale, and as you exhale, bend to your right so that your right elbow is tilting toward the floor.

4. Inhale and return to your starting position.

5. On your next exhale, bend to your left, then lift back up.

6. Repeat this stretch ten times on each side.

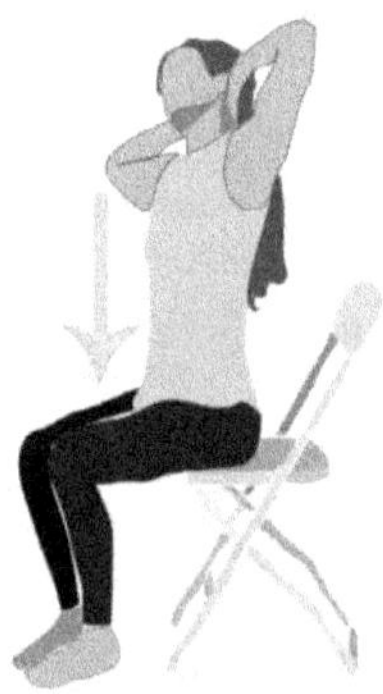

Side stretch

Extended Leg Stretch

1. Sit forward in your chair, keeping your back straight.

2. Extend your left leg out in front of you with your right heel touching the floor and your right toes pointing up toward the ceiling.

3. Keep your left leg bent with your left foot flat on the floor.

4. Inhale, and as you exhale, slowly slide your right hand down your right leg as far as you can go.

5. Slowly return to your starting position.

6. Repeat this stretch ten times on your right side, then switch to your left side.

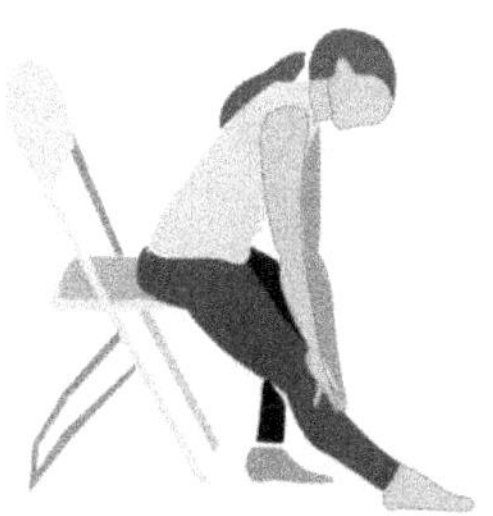

Extended leg stretch

Cross-Legged Stretch

1. Start by sitting slightly forward in an armless chair with your feet flat on the floor and your toes pointing forward. Your hands can rest gently on your thighs.

2. Bend your right knee and place your right ankle on your left knee. It should look like a figure 4. Try to keep your right knee opened out to the side as far as is comfortable.

3. Keeping your back straight, slowly begin to lean forward over your bent leg as you exhale. Stretch as far as you can without any discomfort.

4. Hold here for three breaths, then gently lift back up.

5. Do this 20 times with your right leg, then switch to your left.

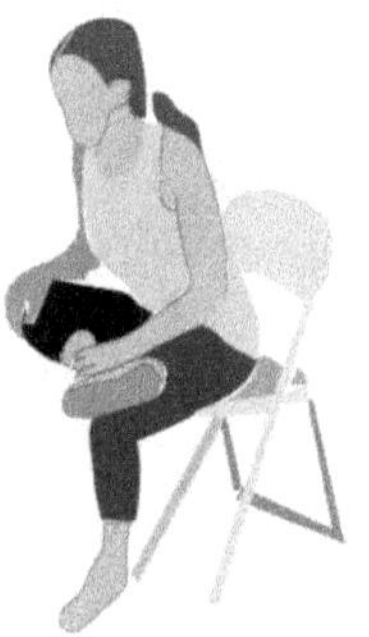

Crossed leg stretch

Side-to-Side Rotation

1. Sit up tall in your chair with your knees hip-width apart and your feet firmly planted on the floor.

2. Cross your arms over your chest.

3. Moving from your waist, turn to the right, then back to center, then to your left and back to center.

4. Keep doing this twist until you have completed ten on each side.

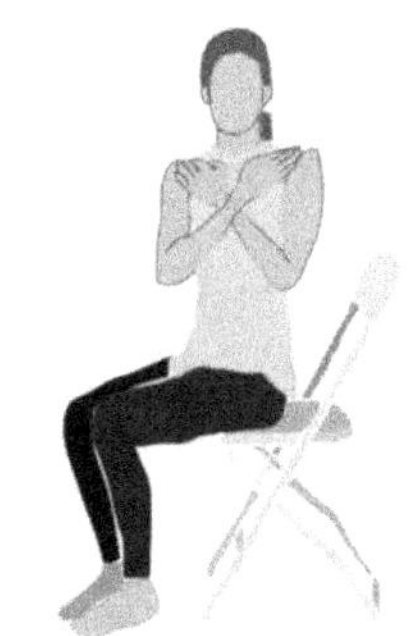

Side to side rotation

Seated Cat-Cow

1. Sit up tall in your chair with your feet firmly on the floor and your knees hip-width apart. Your ankles should be directly under your knees. Your spine should be in a neutral position.

2. Place your hands, palms down, on your knees, with your fingers facing in toward each other.

3. Inhale and lift your chin up toward the ceiling as you arch your back. Keep your shoulders away from your ears.

4. As you exhale, lower your chin to your chest and round your back, pushing your palms into your legs.

5. Repeat this stretch slowly five times.

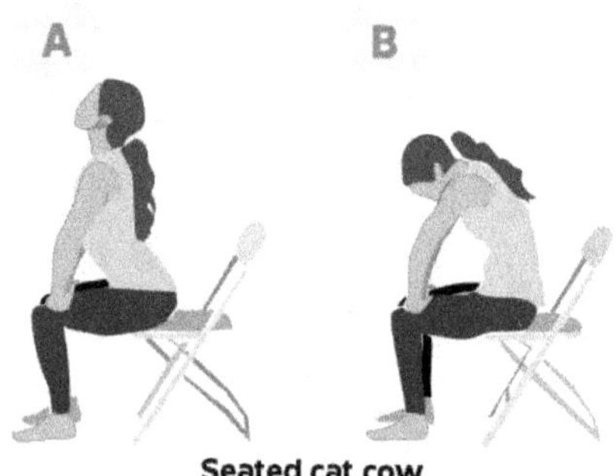

Seated cat cow

Lower Back Stretch

1. Sit forward in your chair with your knees hip-distance apart and your feet pressing into the floor with your toes pointing forward.

2. Place your palms on your lower back with your fingers pointing down.

3. As you inhale, lift your chin up to the ceiling and arch your back slightly. Don't let your head drop too far back.

4. Hold here for one breath, and then exhale, returning to your starting position.

5. Repeat this movement ten times.

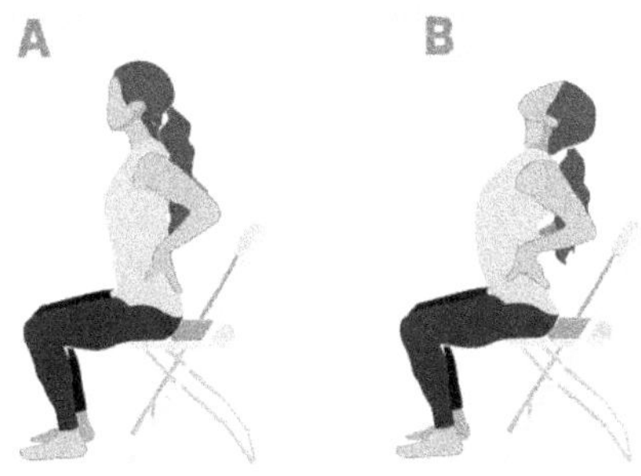
Lower back stretch

Standing Lower Back Stretches

The exercises in this routine can work in conjunction with the previous workout to stretch and lengthen the muscles in the lower back, as well as your legs, in order to give you more strength and stability.

Reaching for the Sky

1. Begin by standing straight with your feet hip-width apart and your toes pointing forward.

2. Lift your arms up and over your head with your palms facing inward. Your arms should be about shoulder-width apart.

3. Hold here for three to five seconds, then release.

4.   Repeat this stretch three times.

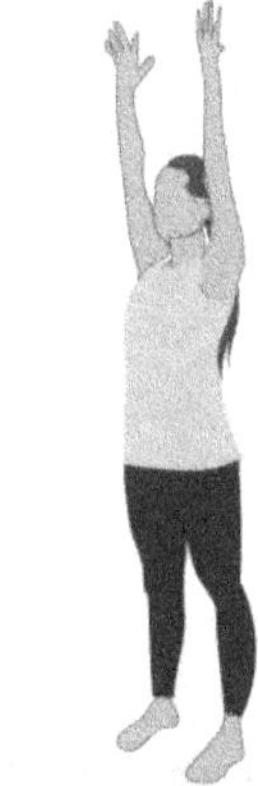

Reaching for the sky

Back Arches

1.   Stand with your feet hip-distance apart and your toes facing forward. Keep a slight bend in your knees.

2.   Place your palms on your lower back with your fingers pointing down.

3.   Slowly lift your chin toward the ceiling, bending your head and upper spine back. You should be able to look up at the ceiling.

4.   Hold here for one to two seconds, then gently lift back up to your starting position.

5.   Repeat this movement three times.

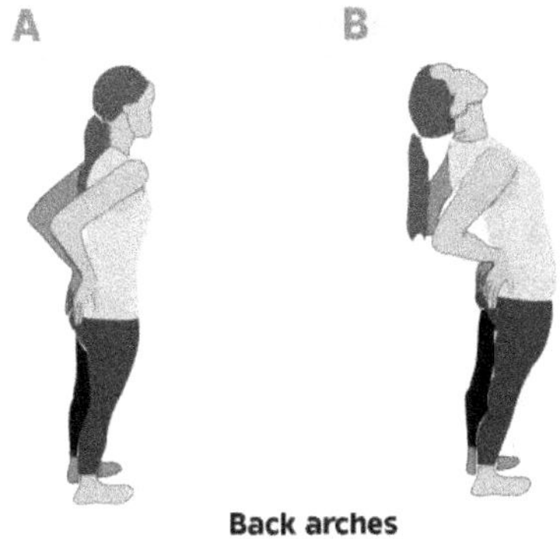

Back arches

Backward Leg Stretch

1.   Stand near a wall or a chair.

2.   Turn so that you can easily hold onto the wall with your right hand.

3.   Place your feet hip-width apart.

4.   Extend your left leg out behind you, keeping your toes on the floor.

5.   Hold here for 20 seconds, then return to your starting position.

6.   Repeat this exercise two times, then switch to the other side.

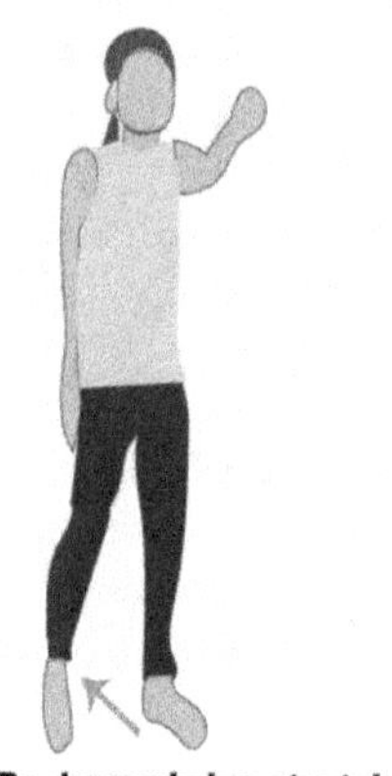

Backwards leg stretch

Leg Swings

1. Using a wall for support, stand sideways so that you can place your right hand on the wall, while keeping your feet hip-width apart.

2. Holding on to the wall, begin to swing your left leg forward and backward.

3. Do this three times in each direction, then turn and repeat with your right leg.

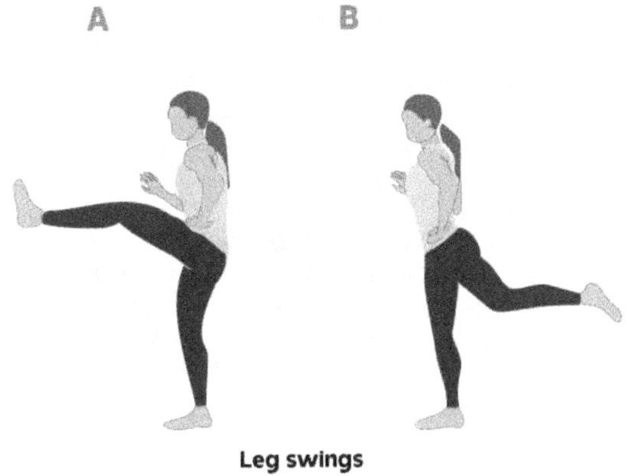

Leg swings

Lower Body Stretch

This lower body stretching routine is a great way to end your workout, as it gives your muscles a chance to recover from all the work they've been doing, and it can help to improve your flexibility. It returns your heart rate and blood pressure to what they were before your activity.

Ankle Pumps

1. Lie down on the floor with your legs extended out and your hands resting at your sides.

2. Slowly flex and point your feet.

3. Repeat this movement 10 to 15 times.

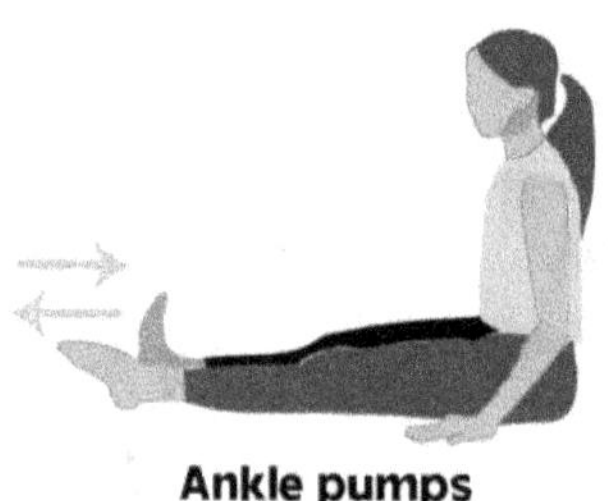

Ankle pumps

Heel Slides

1. Lying on the floor, extend your legs out, keeping them hip-width apart.

2. Place your hands along your sides.

3. Slowly begin to slide your right heel up toward your buttocks, so that your right foot is flat on the floor and your knee is pointing up toward the ceiling.

4. Gently slide the heel back down to your starting position.

5. Repeat this motion 10 to 15 times with your right leg, then repeat with your left leg.

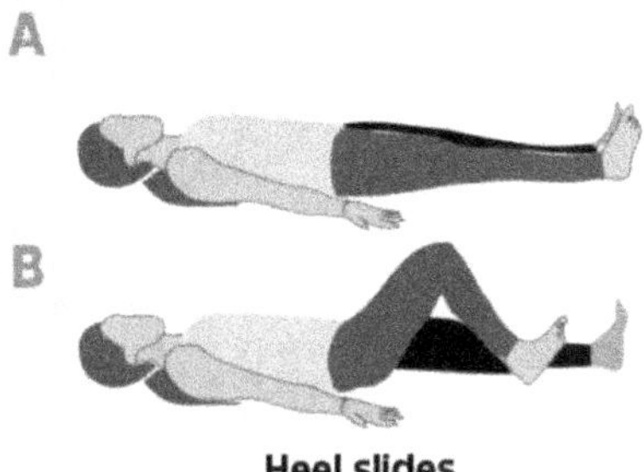

Heel slides

Straight Leg Raise

1. Begin by lying on the floor with your left leg bent so the foot is flat on the floor and the knee is pointing up to the ceiling.

2. Keep your right leg extended out with your toes pointing up.

3. Rest your hands along your sides with your palms facing down.

4. Slowly lift your right leg up, keeping the leg straight, until it is about the height of your left thigh. Then, gently release your leg back to the floor.

5. Do this 10 to 15 times with your right leg, then switch and repeat with your left leg.

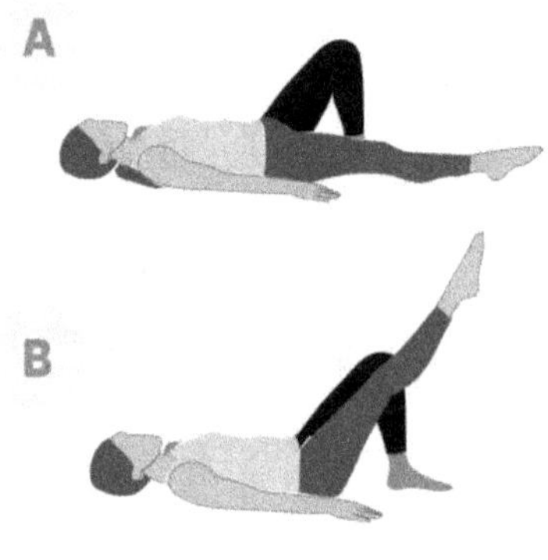

Straight leg raise

Clamshell

1. Lie on your right side with your legs stacked one on top of the other, and your knees bent so your legs are angled behind you.

2. Rest your head on your right arm.

3. Keeping your feet together, raise your left knee up as far as feels comfortable, then gently lower it back down.

4. Repeat this movement 10 to 15 times, then switch to the other side and repeat.

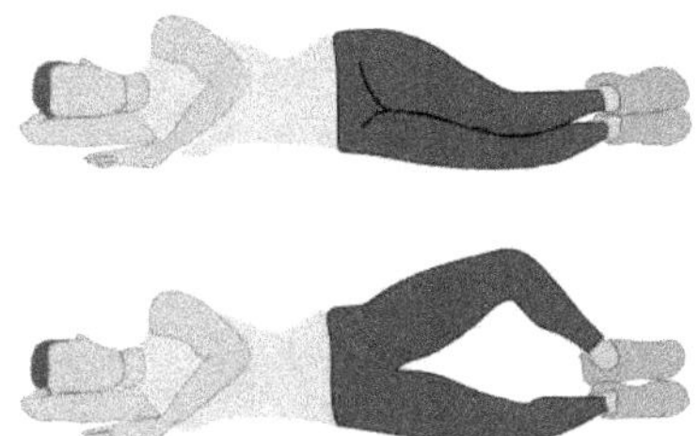

Clamshell

Chapter 6

Healthy Joints for Increased Mobility and Freedom

Basic tasks that we often take for granted like walking, sitting, and lifting require mobility in the knees, hips, wrists, and legs. Joints, especially knee and hip joints, tend to take more impact than is often necessary. This leads to wear and tear on these joints that can result in pain and reduced mobility.

As we get older, we are also more prone to inflammation and swelling of our joints, as well as the breakdown of cartilage around the joints. Hip pain can be a direct result of weakened hip muscles, usually associated with a lack of movement. All of these can be extremely painful and increase our risk of falls and injuries.

These ailments can be managed or prevented by maintaining a healthy weight and regular, daily exercise. Excess weight can increase the pressure on our joints and ligaments, making it more difficult to move and perform our daily tasks. By exercising, you can maintain your weight as well as stretch and strengthen the muscles surrounding your joints.

Strong hip muscles increase the stability of your knees and therefore lowers the risk of knee pain or injury. Stretching and exercising the elbows and wrists increases the production of synovial fluid (thick liquid between the joints), which results in better lubrication of the joints, helping to improve their function.

The exercises in this section target the joints to help increase mobility and to ensure that you can enjoy your independence for a long time to come.

Hip Strengthening

The muscles in our hips provide stability to our lower body and protect our spine. Strengthening these muscles will help to reduce hip pain and prevent problems with posture as well as balance.

Butterfly Pose

1. Sit on the floor with your back straight and your shoulders down away from your ears.

2. Bring the soles of your feet together to touch, opening your knees in the shape of a butterfly.

3. Sitting up tall, hold your ankles with your hands.

4. Inhale, and as you exhale, slowly lean your upper body forward until you feel a stretch. The closer your heels are to your body, the more you will stretch the hip muscles, but this takes time.

5. Try to keep your knees pressed down, and do not lift up off your seat.

6. Hold here for five seconds, then lift back up. Repeat ten times.

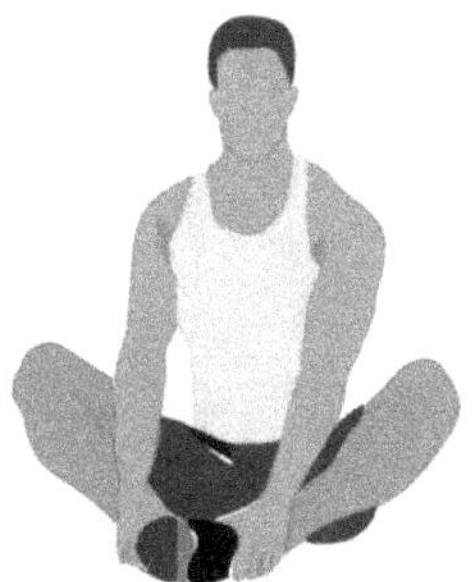

Butterfly pose

Standing Hip Flexor

1. Begin by standing with your feet hip-width apart and your hands on your hips.

2. Step your right foot forward and slowly bend your left knee as you lift your left heel off the floor.

3. Use a chair or wall to keep your balance as you hold for five seconds.

4. Slowly come back to standing.

5. Repeat this movement with your left leg.

6. You can do this exercise three times on each side.

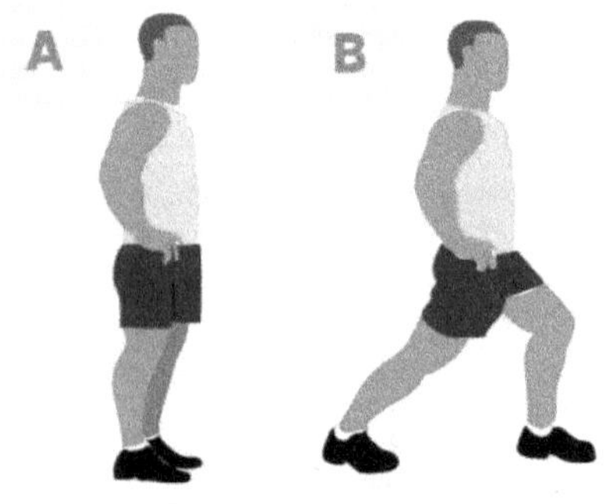

Standing hip flexor

Standing Hip Extension With Chair Support

1. Stand straight with your arms at your sides and your shoulders wide. Keep a chair or table in front of you for support.

2. Keeping your hands on the chair, extend your right leg back with your toes touching the ground.

3. Return to your starting position.

4. Do this exercise ten times on your right leg, then switch to your left.

5. If the movement seems too easy, you can add some ankle weights for more resistance.

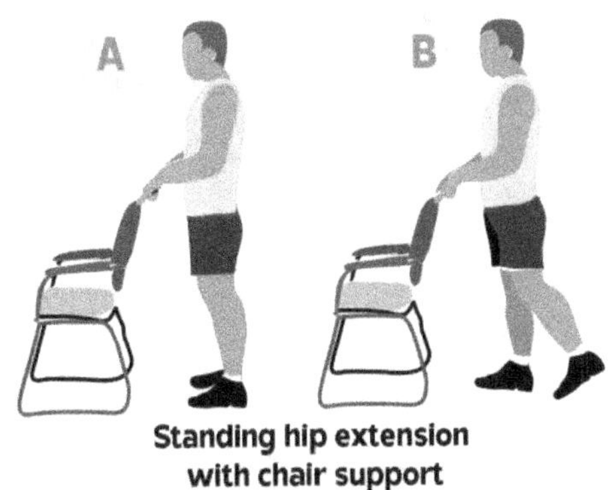

**Standing hip extension
with chair support**

Side Hip Raises

1. Come to lie on your right side on the floor with your legs extended and stacked one on top of the other. You can use a pillow to cushion your head if it feels more comfortable.

2. Place your left hand in front of you for support as you lift your left leg up. Only go as far as feels good to you.

3. Slowly lower your left leg down to meet your right.

4. Repeat this movement five times with your left leg, then switch to your right.

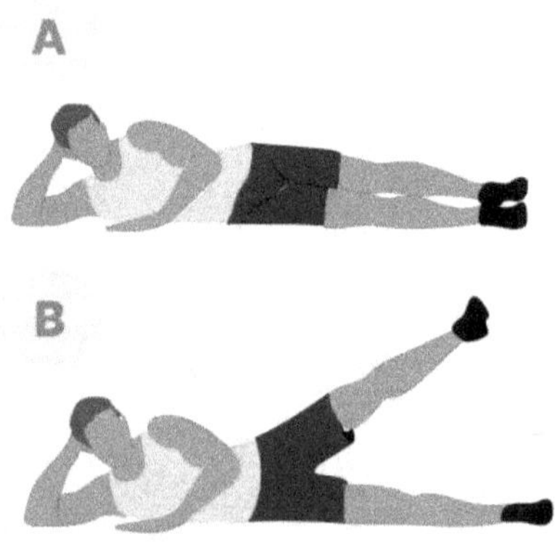

Side hip raise

Straight Leg Raises

1. Begin by lying face down on the floor.

2. Using the muscles of your stomach, slowly lift your right leg up.

3. Hold for three seconds, then gently lower down.

4. Repeat this movement five times with each leg.

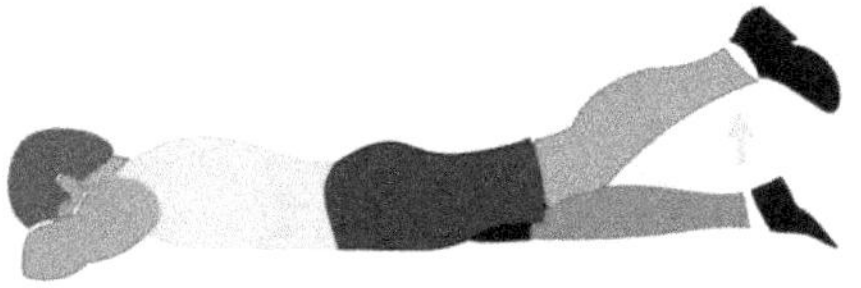

Straight leg raise

Standing Hip Abductors With Chair Support

1. Stand tall with a wall or chair in front of you for support.

2. Holding on to the chair, slowly lift your right leg backward off the ground and hold for three seconds.

3. Make a half circle with your extended leg, then return your right foot back to the ground.

4. Repeat this exercise five times with your right leg, then switch to your left.

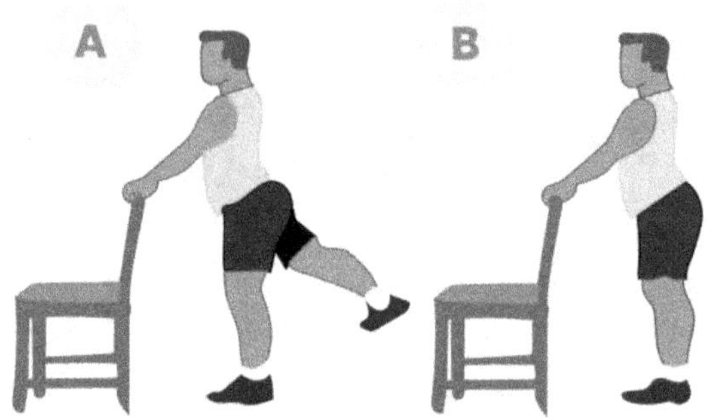

**Standing hip abductions
with chair support**

Hip Circles

1. Begin by standing straight with your feet slightly wider that shoulder-distance apart.

2. Place your hands on your hips and bend your knees a bit.

3. Moving in a clockwise direction, slowly rotate your hips, making a big circle, and keeping your feet firmly pressed into the ground.

4. Move in this direction for about 30 seconds, then reverse your circles, going for another 30 seconds.

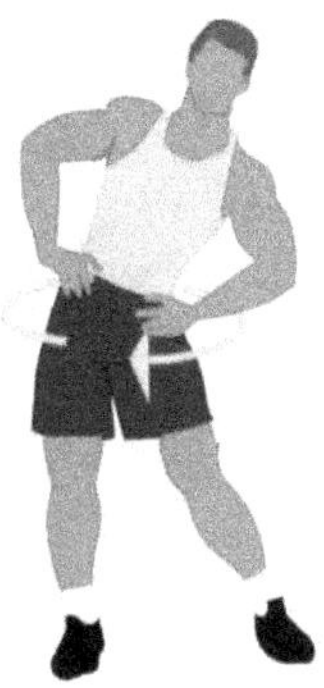

Hip circles

Seated Hip Marches

1. Sit up tall in an unpadded chair with your feet flat on the floor. Make sure your back is against the chair so that you can keep a proper posture.

2. Place your hands lightly on your thighs.

3. Lift your right knee as high as is comfortable, then lower it back to the floor.

4. Alternate with your left knee as if you were marching on the spot.

5. Try to do at least 10 to 15 lifts with each leg.

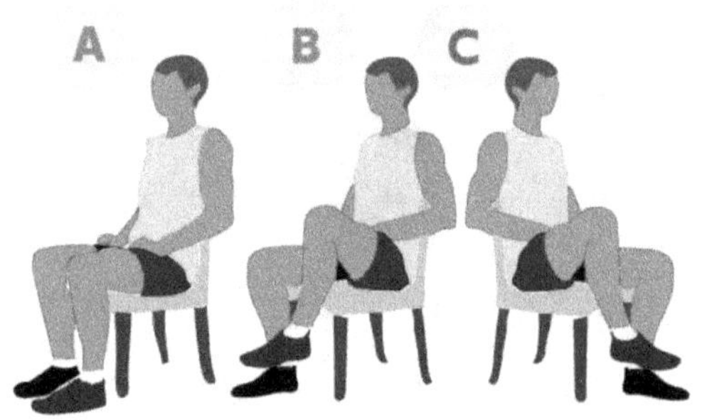

Seated hip marches

Knee-to-Chest

1. Begin by lying on your back on the floor with your legs extended.

2. Slowly bring your right knee up to your chest, as close as you can get it, and wrap your arms around your right knee, hugging it to your chest.

3. Hold for 20 seconds, then slowly release your right leg back to the floor.

4. Repeat this with your left leg. Do this exercise three times with each leg.

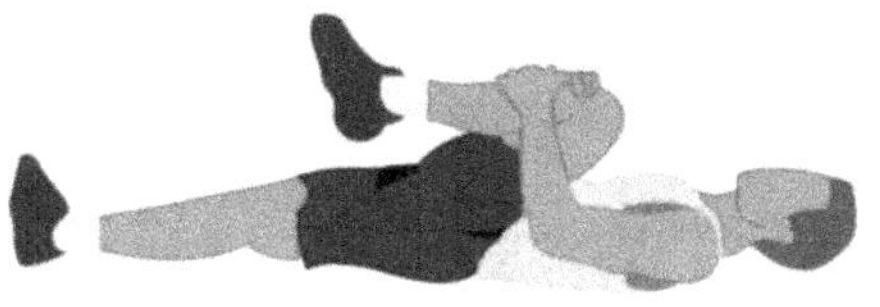

Knee Strengthening

Our knees are constantly under pressure from walking, standing, and moving in general. This routine is meant to aid you in strengthening the muscles and tendons that support your knees. In turn, this ensures that you can move more confidently with less risk of falling and injury.

Calf Raises

1. Begin by standing on a step or a stool with your heels hanging off the edge slightly. Be sure to have something to hold on to for balance.

2. Slowly rise up on your toes, letting your heels come up. You should feel the muscles in your calf working and flexing.

3. Gently lower back down, letting your heels go a little past the level of the step.

4. Repeat these calf raises ten times for a maximum of three sets.

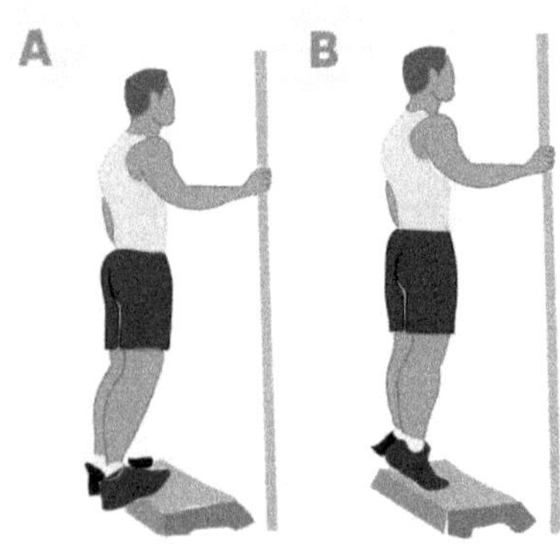

Calf raises

Seated Knee Extensions

1. Sit up straight in an unpadded chair with your feet flat on the floor.

2. Lift your right knee up and extend your right leg out in front of you while staying seated. Hold, and then lower back down.

3. Now repeat this movement with your right leg.

4. Repeat these knee extensions ten times on each leg for a maximum of three sets.

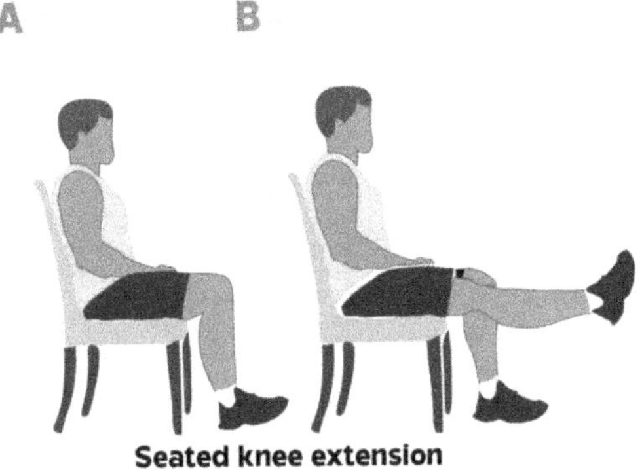

Seated knee extension

Standing Knee Flex With Chair Support

1. Start by standing with a chair in front of you for support.

2. Lift your left foot off the floor behind you, bending at the knee. Go as far as feels comfortable.

3. Repeat this movement ten times with your left leg, then switch to your right.

4. You can do up to three sets on each side.

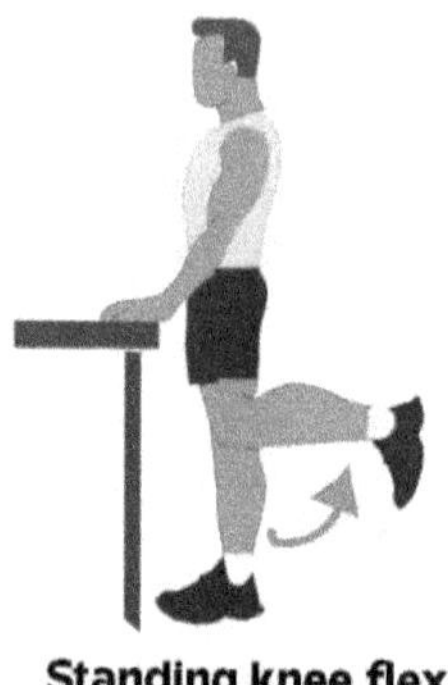

**Standing knee flex
with chair support**

Reclined Leg Lifts

1. Begin by lying on the floor with your legs straight out.

2. Bend your left knee and place your left foot on the floor with your knee pointing up toward the ceiling.

3. Keeping your right leg extended, lift it up as high as you can, then lower it slowly to the floor.

4. Do this movement ten times with your right leg, then switch and complete it with your left leg.

5. You can try to do three sets on each side.

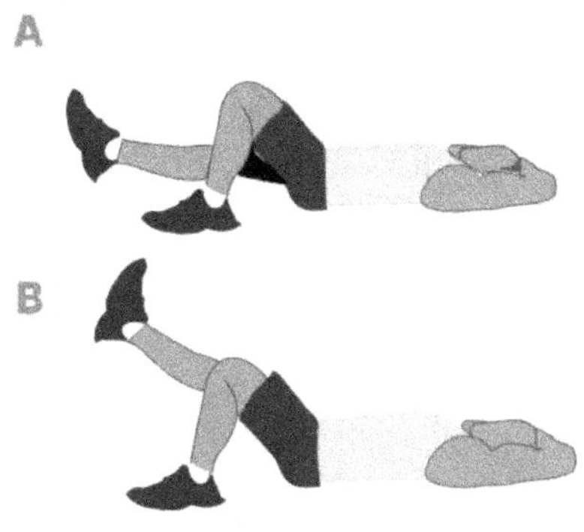

Reclined leg lifts

Wall Squats

1. Stand with your back against a wall, with your feet hip-width apart, and your arms at your sides.

2. Slowly begin to lower yourself by bending your knees while keeping your back against the wall. Be sure to keep your knees in line with your feet, and your back with your pelvis.

3. Hold this squat for three to ten seconds, then slide back up to standing, making sure to keep your back against the wall.

4. Repeat this exercise ten times for up to three sets, depending on how you feel.

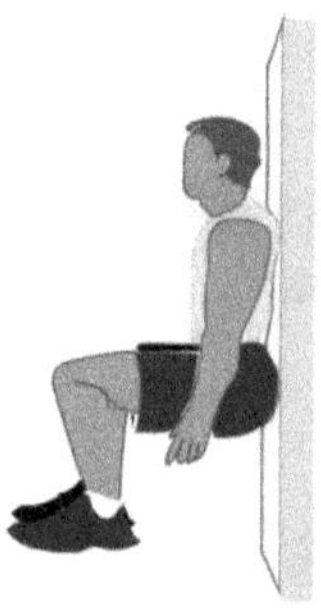

Wall squats

Step Ups

1. Stand up tall in front of a step or workout stool. You can use a chair for balance if you need it.

2. With your right foot, step up onto the step, then your left.

3. Step down with your right foot, then your left.

4. Repeat these movements ten times for up to three sets. Change the foot you start with on every other set.

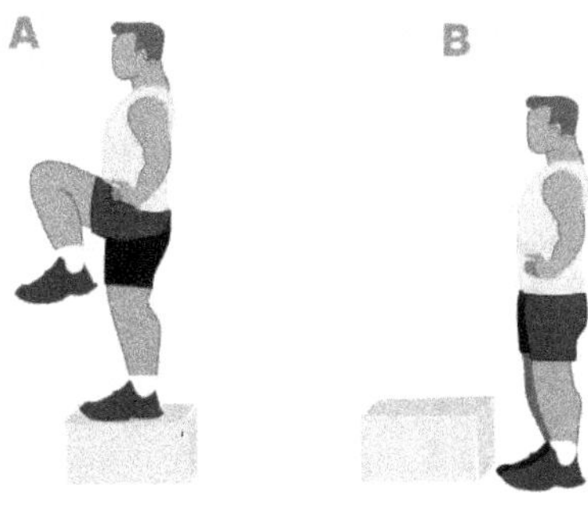

Step ups

Side Steps

1. Stand with your feet hip-distance apart and your arms relaxed at your sides.

2. Step wide to your right with your right foot, then bring your left foot to meet your right one.

3. Now step wide with your left foot, then bring your right foot to meet your left foot.

4. Continue doing this ten times for up to three sets.

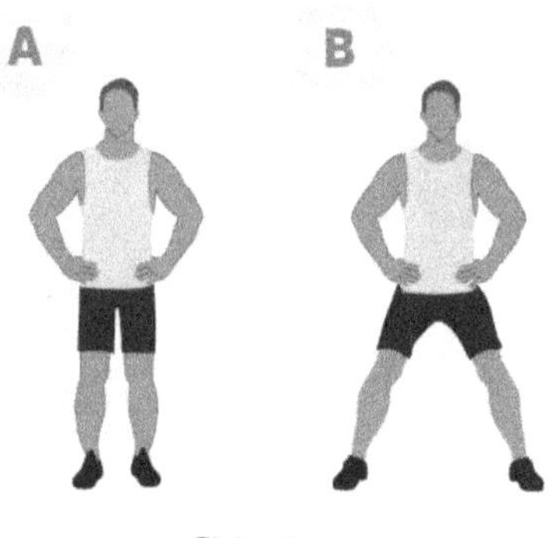

Side steps

Clamshell

1. Lie on your right side with your legs stacked one on top of the other at a 45-degree angle. Rest your head on your right arm, or you can bend your right arm at the elbow and prop your head on your hand.

2. Keeping your feet together, raise your left knee up to the ceiling, going only as far as feels comfortable.

3. Gently lower your left knee back down to touch the right.

4. Do this exercise ten times on the right, then switch over to your left. You can repeat on each side for up to three sets.

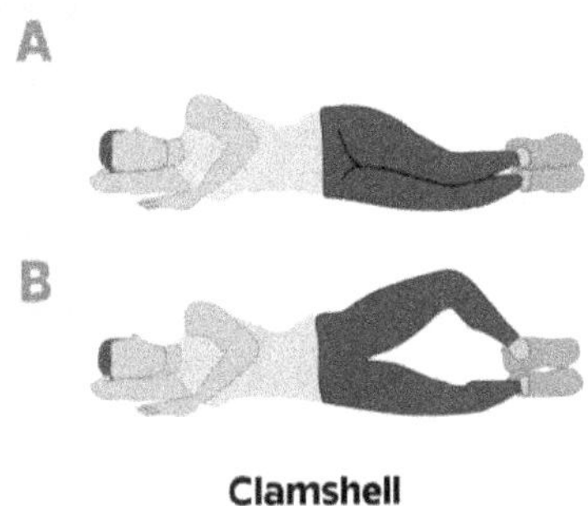

Clamshell

Elbow Strengthening

This routine focuses on your arm muscles, which you need for picking up groceries, reaching items off shelves, and for daily self-care. The goal of this workout is to make sure you can do your daily tasks independently. For these exercises, you will require dumbbells between one and five pounds.

Shoulder Rolls

1. Sit up comfortably in a chair with weights in both hands and your arms extended down along your sides.

2. Lift your shoulders up, back, and then down.

3. Repeat these rolls ten times in this direction, then switch to the opposite direction for ten more repetitions.

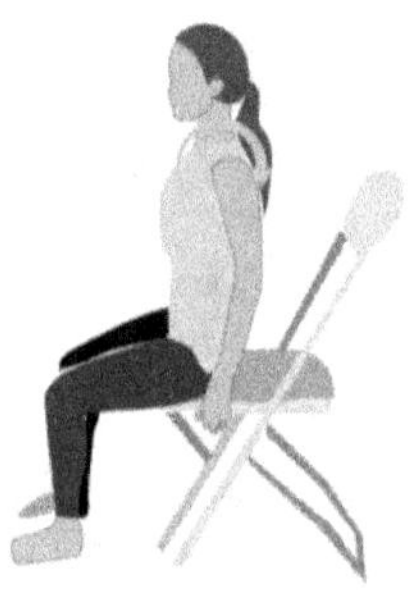

Seated shoulder roll

Seated Bicep Curls

1. Sit in a chair with no arms, making sure that your back is straight against the chair back and your feet are flat on the floor.

2. Hold the weight in your right hand with your palm facing inward.

3. Bend your elbow up toward your shoulder as you turn your palm up.

4. Slowly lower your arm back to the starting position.

5. Repeat this movement ten times with your right arm, then switch the weight over to your left hand and do another ten repetitions.

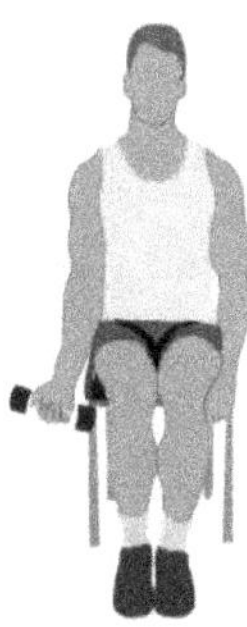

Seated bicep curl

Seated Overhead Elbow Extension

1. Begin by sitting in a chair with your back flush against the chair back and your feet flat on the floor.

2. Hold the weight in your right hand and lift your right arm up, keeping your elbow bent. Your elbow should be pointing up toward the ceiling.

3. Slowly straighten your elbow, lifting your right hand above your head.

4. Lower your right hand back to your starting position with your elbow pointing up.

5. Repeat this movement eight times on your right side, then switch to your left.

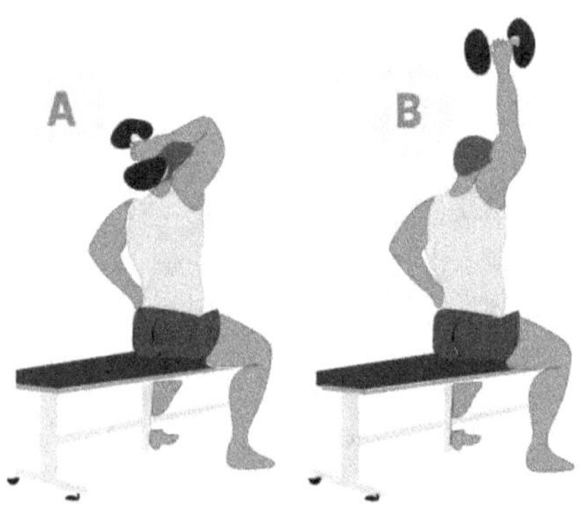

Seated overhead elbow extension

Triceps Kickbacks With Chair Support

1. Start by placing a chair in front you for support.

2. Hold the weight in your right hand and bend your elbow so your arm is close to your chest. Place your left hand on the back of the chair and lean over the chair.

3. As you inhale, slowly extend your right arm out behind you as far as feels comfortable, then return to your starting position as you exhale.

4. Repeat this movement eight times with your right arm, then switch to your left for eight more repetitions.

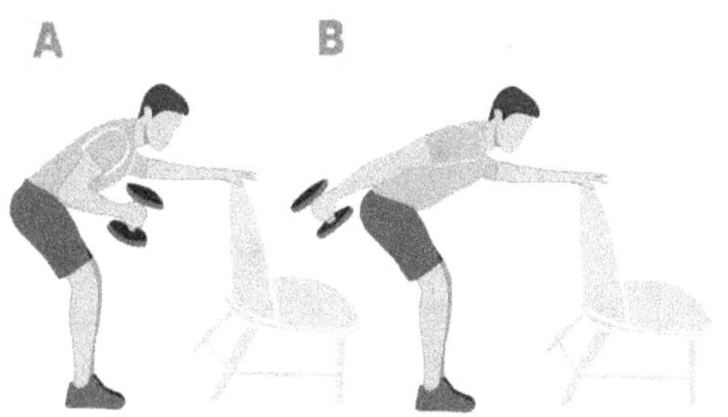

Triceps kickback with chair support

Seated Diagonal Inward Shoulder Raise

1. Sit in a chair with no arms with your back straight against the chair back and your feet flat on the floor.

2. Place the weight in your right hand with the palm facing forward and your arm extended down to your side. Keep your left hand on your left thigh.

3. Inhale and slowly lift your right arm up and across your body to your left shoulder, bending your elbow and turning the palm to face inward.

4. Exhale while returning to your starting position.

5. Repeat this exercise eight times on your right side, then switch to your left.

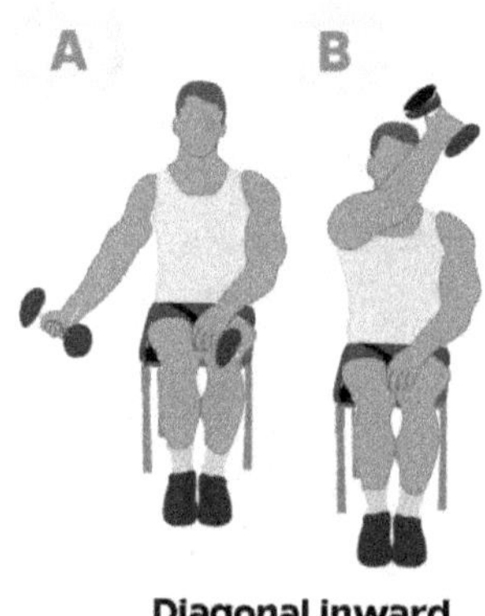

**Diagonal inward
shoulder raise**

Seated Diagonal Outward Shoulder Raise

1. Begin by sitting up straight in a chair with no arms and your feet flat on the floor.

2. Hold a weight in your right hand and cross your right arm over your body so that the weight is near your left hip. Keep your right palm facing in and your left arm at your side.

3. Inhale and lift your right arm up and across your body, ending with your arm extended up to your right side with the palm facing out.

4. Exhale and return to your starting position.

5. Repeat this movement eight times on your right side, then move to your left side.

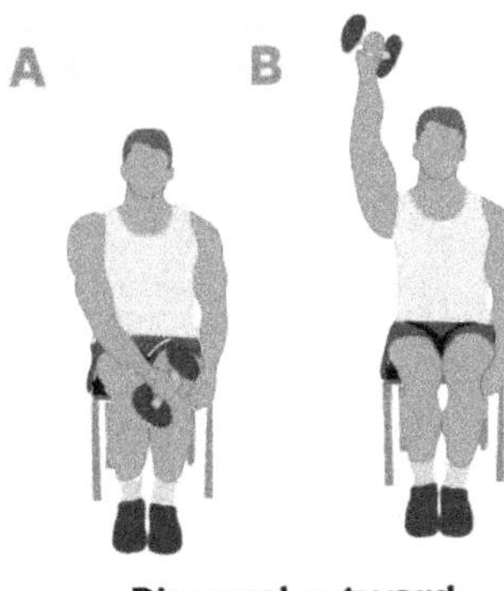

Diagonal outward shoulder raise

Seated Overhead Press

1. Sit in a chair with your feet shoulder-distance apart and weights in both hands.

2. Open your arms out to the side, keeping your elbows bent so that your weights are at shoulder-level and your palms are facing out.

3. Inhale and extend your arms straight above your head.

4. Exhale and return to your starting position.

5. Repeat this exercise ten times.

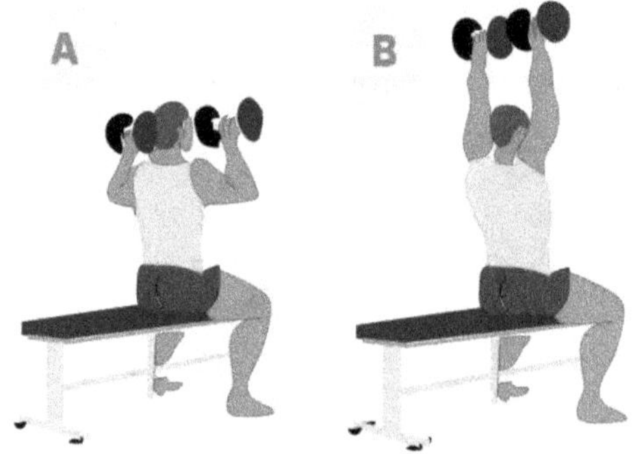

Seated overhead press

Reclined Shoulder Press

1. Lie on the floor on your back, making sure that your head, back, and buttocks are firmly pressed into the floor.

2. Hold weights in both hands with your arms bent at 90 degrees on either side of you.

3. As you inhale, extend your arms up toward the ceiling with your palms facing each other.

4. Exhale and lower to your starting position.

5. Repeat this movement ten times.

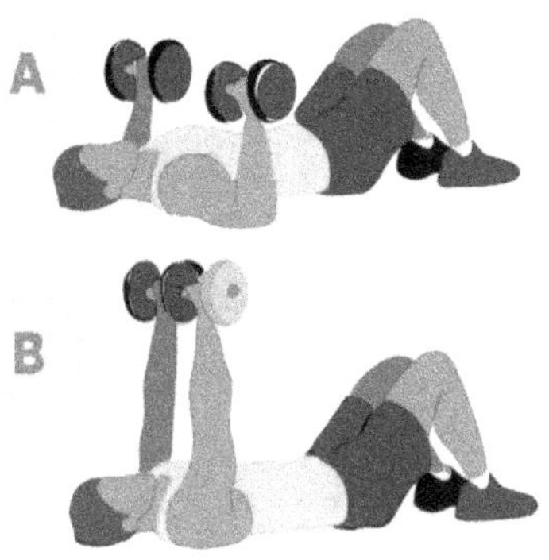

Reclined shoulder press

Upright Rows

1. Stand with your feet shoulder-distance apart. Hold weights in both your hands in front of your hips with your palms facing in, toward your body.

2. Inhale as you lift the weights up toward your chin, as if you were sliding them up your chest.

3. Exhale, and lower the weights back down to your hips.

4. Repeat this exercise eight times.

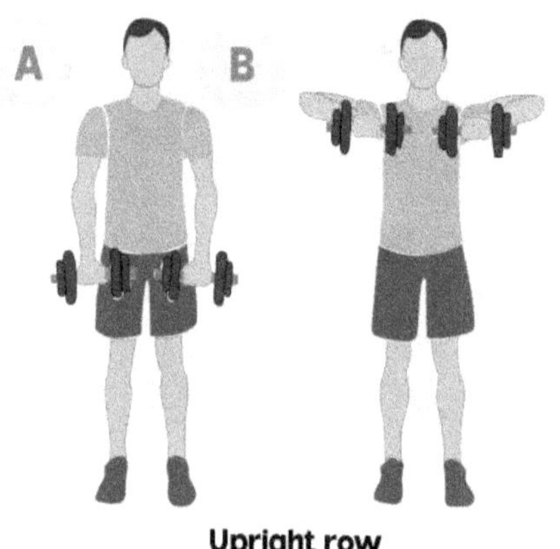

Upright row

Bent Over Rows

1. Place a chair in front of you and lean over it, placing your left hand on the chair back for stability.

2. Hold a weight in your right hand with your palm facing in.

3. Inhale and lift your arm up behind you, bending your elbow so that it comes to shoulder height.

4. Exhale and lower your arm back down.

5. Repeat this movement eight times on your right side, then move to your left side and do eight more repetitions.

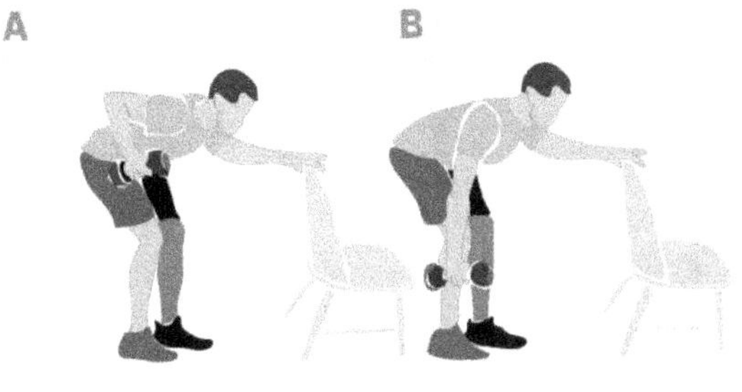

Bent over row

Side Shoulder Lifts

1. Stand with your feet hip-width apart and your arms extended down at your sides, with your elbows straight.

2. Hold a weight in your right hand with the palm facing forward.

3. As you inhale, lift your right arm out to the side and up toward the ceiling.

4. Exhale as you lower your arm back to your side.

5. Repeat this movement eight times with your right arm, then switch to your left.

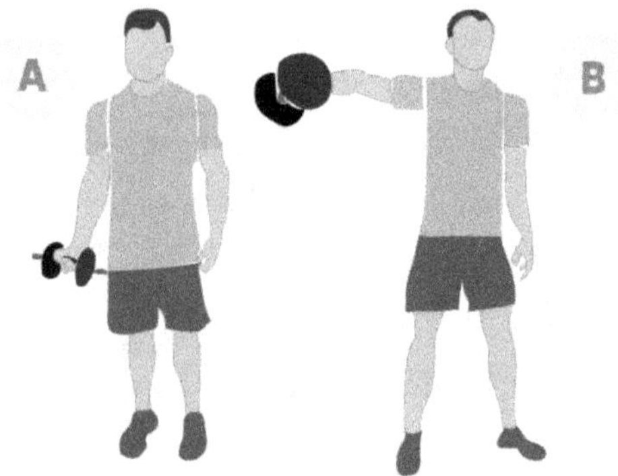

Side shoulder lift

Elbow Side Extensions

1. Stand with your feet shoulder-distance apart and flat on the floor.

2. Hold weights in both hands in front of your chest with your elbows bent up and out to either side and your palms facing in toward your chest.

3. On an inhale, open your arms out to either side with your palms facing forward.

4. Exhale and return to your starting position.

5. Repeat this exercise eight times.

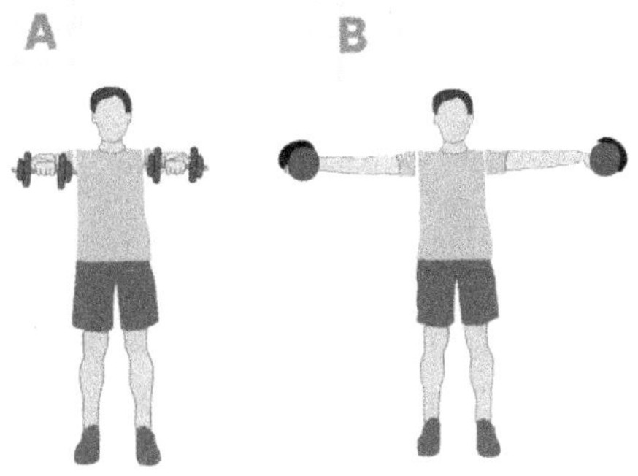

Elbow side extension

Wrist and Hand Strengthening

Stretching and exercising your wrists and hands increase the production of synovial fluid, which lubricates the joints around these areas, making it easier to use and move them, regardless of pain or discomfort. These exercises help to keep your wrists and hands strong and flexible therefore prevent injury.

Wrist Warm-Up

1. Sit comfortably with your feet flat on the floor. Bend your right arm at the elbow and use your left hand to support your right arm at the elbow.

2. Make a fist with your right hand and slowly flex the wrist up as far as you can, and then down as far as feels comfortable.

3. Repeat this up and down movement ten times.

4. Now, keeping your hand in the same starting position, move your right wrist left to right as far as it can go without causing any discomfort. Try not to move your arm, just your wrist.

5. Repeat this left to right movement ten times.

6. Switch hands and repeat both movements with your left hand.

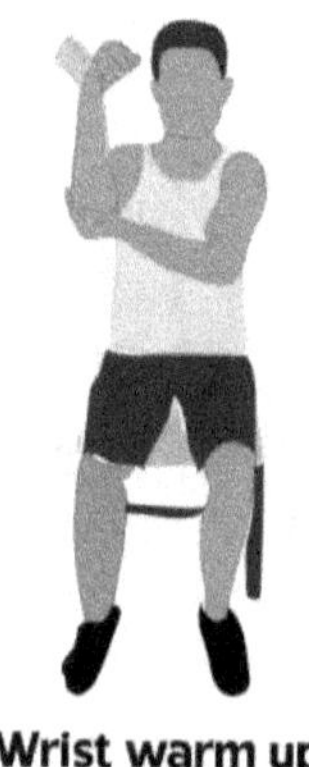

Wrist warm up

Wrist Lifts With Palms Down

1. Sit up tall in a chair with your feet flat on the floor.

2. Place your hands on your thighs with your palms facing down.

3. With your fingers outstretched, raise them toward the ceiling, moving only your wrists. Be sure to keep the heels of your palms on your thighs.

4. Lower your fingers back down.

5. Repeat this movement five times for up to three sets.

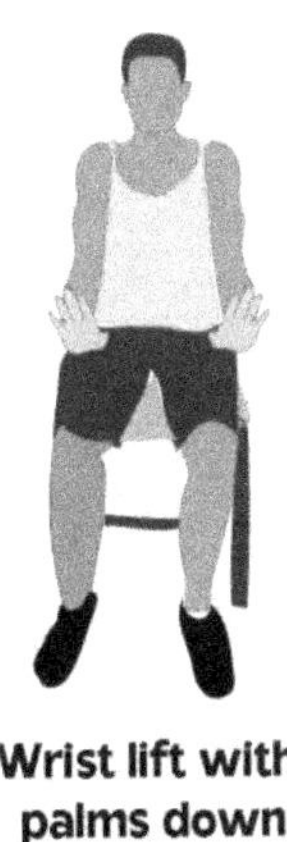

Wrist lift with palms down

Wrist Lifts With Palms Up

1. Sit up tall in a chair with your feet flat on the floor.

2. Place your hands on your thighs with your palms facing up.

3. With your fingers outstretched, raise them toward the ceiling, moving only your wrists. Be sure to keep the heels of your palms on your thighs and only go as far as feels comfortable.

4. Lower your fingers back down.

5. Repeat this movement five times for up to three sets.

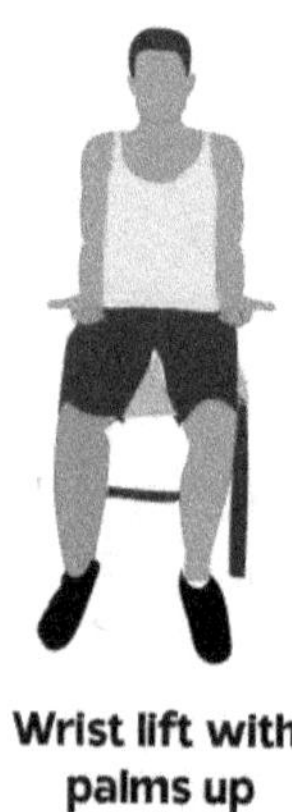

Wrist lift with palms up

Finger Stretches

1. Sit with your right elbow bent at a 90 degree angle.

2. Make a fist with your right hand, then slowly open your fingers, spreading and stretching them as far apart as you can.

3. Repeat this open and close movement three times with your right hand, then switch to your left hand and repeat.

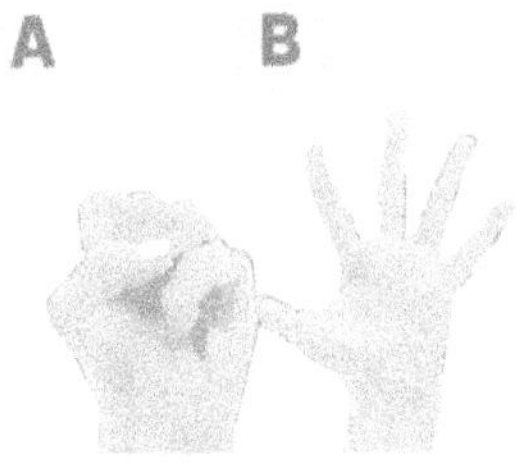

Finger stretches

Prayer Stretch

1. Stand with your feet hip-width apart and your hands in prayer position just below your chin, with your elbows close to your sides.

2. Keeping your hands pressed firmly together, lower your hands toward your waist until you feel a stretch in your forearms. Keep your hands close to your body.

3. Hold for 30 seconds, then return to your starting prayer position.

4. Repeat this movement up to four times.

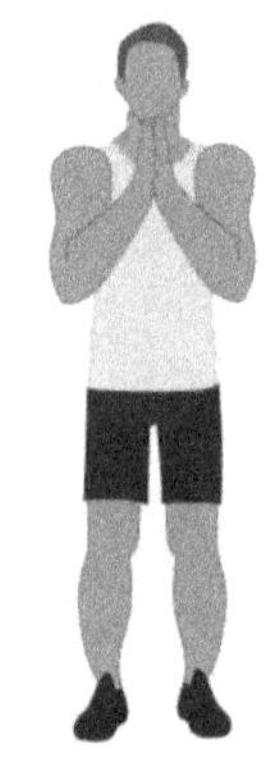

Prayer stretch

Steeple Prayer Stretch

1. Stand with your hands in a prayer position with your fingers just under your chin.

2. Keeping your hands firmly pressed together, spread your fingers and thumbs as far apart as you can.

3. Now move your palms away from each other, but keep your fingers and thumbs pressing together. Return your palms to touch again.

4. Repeat this exercise up to four times.

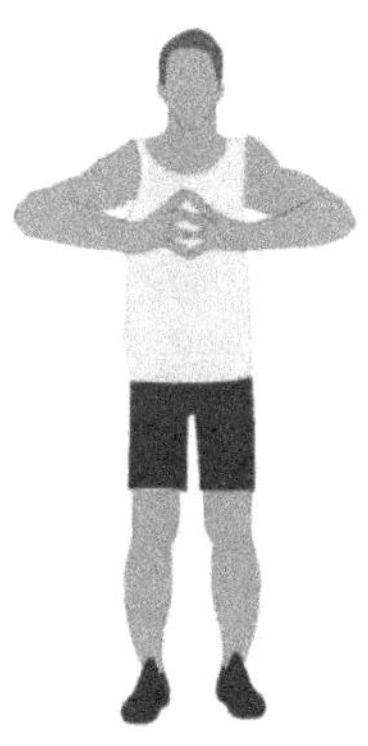

Steeple stretch

Hand Strengthening Ball Squeeze

1. Sitting comfortably, hold a ball (a tennis ball, or something of a similar size) in your right hand, making sure to wrap your fingers and thumb firmly around it.

2. Squeeze the ball as hard as you can for about three to five seconds, then relax your grip.

3. Repeat this exercise five to ten times with your right hand, then move the ball to your left hand and do the same thing.

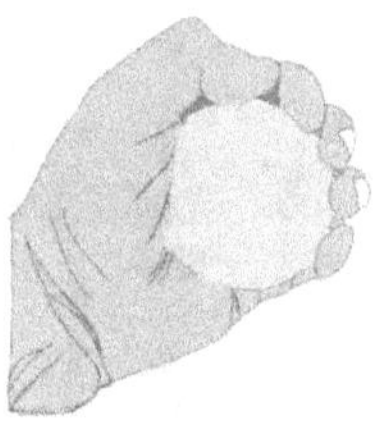

**Hand strengthening
ball squeeze**

Rubber Band Strengthener

1. Sitting comfortably, stretch a rubber band around the tops of your right fingers and thumb.

2. Slowly open your hand, stretching the rubber band as far as you can, then slowly close your fingers. Try to control your movements.

3. Repeat this exercise five to ten times with your right hand, then switch to your left.

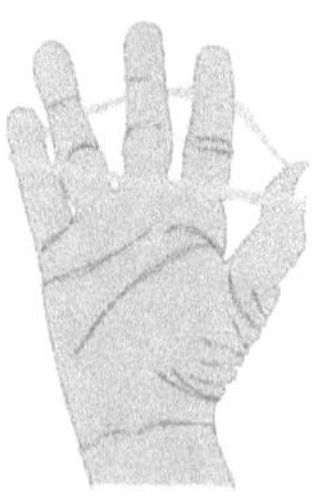

Rubber band strengthener

Wrist Curls

1. Sit straight in a chair with your feet flat on the
    floor.

2. Rest your arms on your knees with your wrists
    hanging over them.

3. Either make a fist or hold a weight with your
    right hand, but keep your palm facing down.

4. Move your right hand up and then down as far
    as it will comfortably go. Keep your movements
    slow and controlled.

5. Repeat this movement ten times for up to three
    sets.

6. Once you've finished on your right side, move
    over to your left hand and repeat.

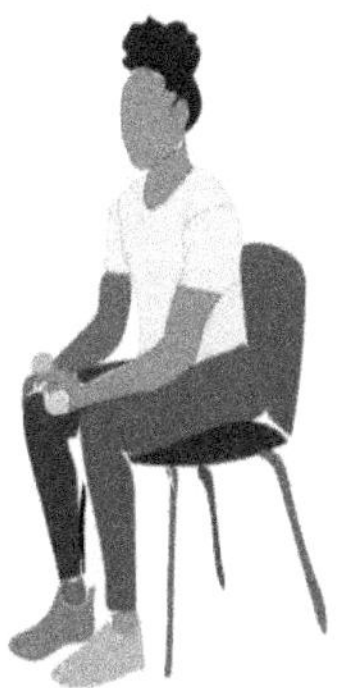

Wrist curls

Wrist Walking

1. Stand facing a wall with your hands extended out in front of you, and your palms pressed against the wall, with your fingers pointing up toward the ceiling.

2. With your palms firmly pressing against the wall, walk your wrists down the wall as far as they can go without your palms lifting off.

3. Now, turn your hands so that your fingers are pointing down.

4. Once again, keep your palms against the wall, and now walk your wrists back up the wall as far as they can go.

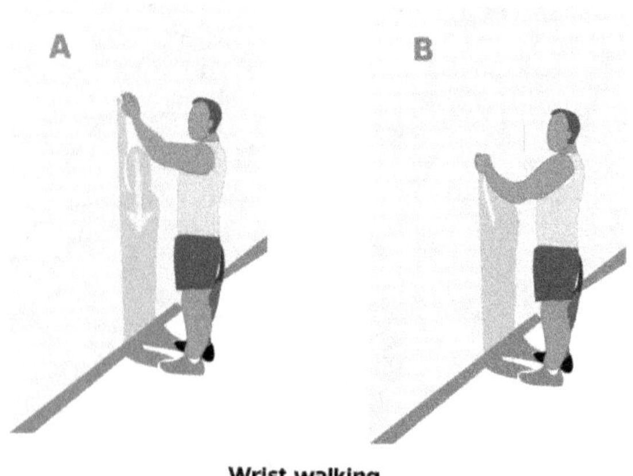

Wrist walking

Grip Strengthening

1. Sit comfortably with your right arm bent at a 90 degree angle.

2. Hold a gripper or soft ball in your right hand with your palm facing inward.

3. Slowly squeeze the gripper or ball, then release it. Try to move only your hand, not your arm.

4. Repeat this movement ten times for up to three sets.

5. Switch and repeat with your left hand.

6. You can use a gripper with more tension as you become more comfortable with this exercise.

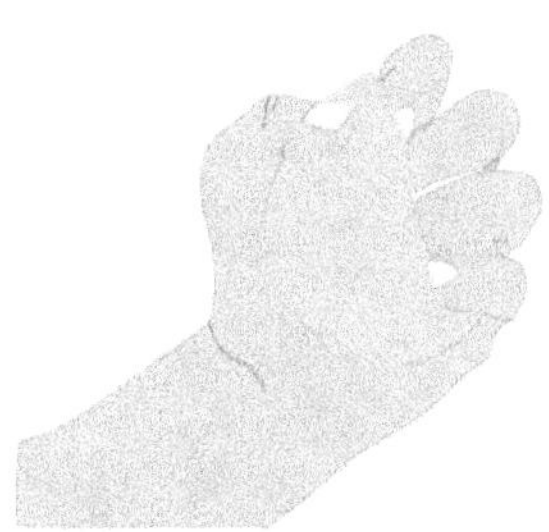

Grip strengthening

Chapter 7:

Why Lower Body Exercises

Are Crucial

Our largest muscles are found in our lower body, and as a result, our lower body is the foundation for most activities like walking, jumping, bending, or dancing. In fact, our entire body is stabilized by our lower body. As such, focusing on our lower body can help us to maintain strength and prevent strains, sprains, and fractures.

Our glutes and butt muscles are responsible for moving our upper legs to the side and back, while our abductors move our legs to the side and back to the midline. Our hamstrings raise our heels toward our buttocks and our quadriceps are responsible for straightening the leg, extending the knee, and helping us to lift. If these muscles are weak, then we are at great risk of injuries, as well as more prone to pain as we age.

Ensuring that we maintain strength in our lower body as we get older is integral to ensuring our continued independence and overall health. Regular lower body exercise can improve your balance and increase bone strength, a definite asset as we age. This, in turn, lowers your risk of falling and of sustaining knee or hip injuries. It also raises your energy levels and lowers your pain levels. An even greater side effect of a strong lower body is that it boosts your confidence in yourself and in your ability to lead a healthy, independent life.

Foot and Ankle Exercises

Your feet and ankles are critical in helping you to maintain your balance and stability. If the muscles in these areas are weak, then chances are you will experience pain or discomfort and you can increase your risk of falling and injury. This routine focuses on building and maintaining strength in your ankles and feet in order to better support you.

Ankle Circles Warm-Up

1. Begin by sitting all the way back on a sturdy chair with your feet flat on the floor.

2. Extend your right leg out in front of you and begin to rotate your ankle in a clockwise direction.

3. Repeat 20 times in this direction, then rotate your right ankle in a counterclockwise motion 20 more times.

4. When you're finished on your right leg, move to your left leg and repeat the same movements.

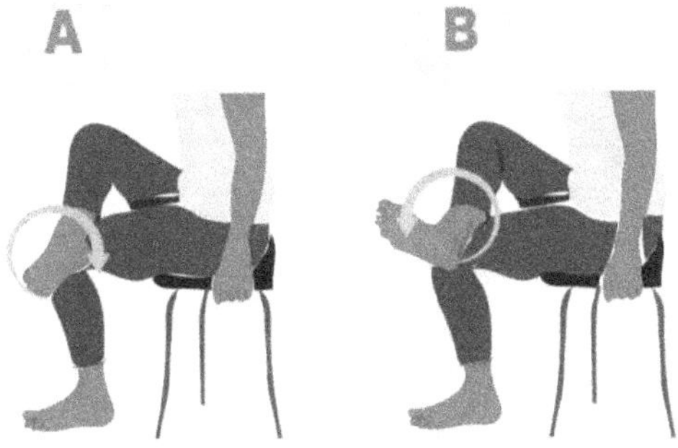

Ankle circles

Heel Raises

1. Begin by standing behind a chair and holding on to the back rest for support, but try not to lean into it.

2. As you exhale, raise your heels off the floor as far as feels comfortable.

3. Take three deep breaths with your heels lifted.

4. On your next inhale, lower your heels back to the ground.

5. Repeat this movement ten times.

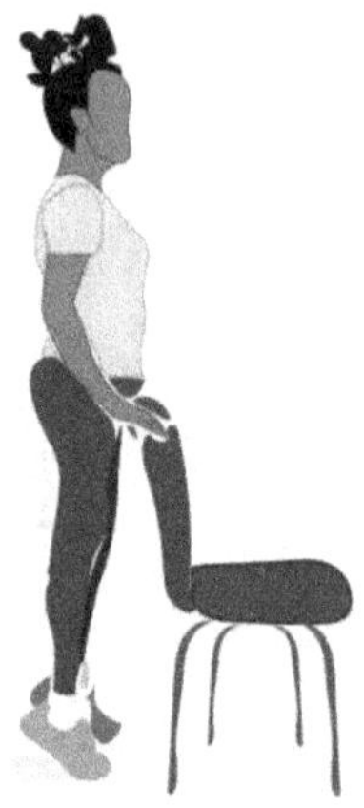

Heel raises

Butt Squeezes

1. You can begin this exercise either by sitting up or lying down. Choose whichever is more comfortable or more convenient for you.

2. Once you're ready, tighten your butt cheeks as if you're trying to squeeze them together.

3. Hold for three seconds, then relax.

4. Repeat this motion ten times.

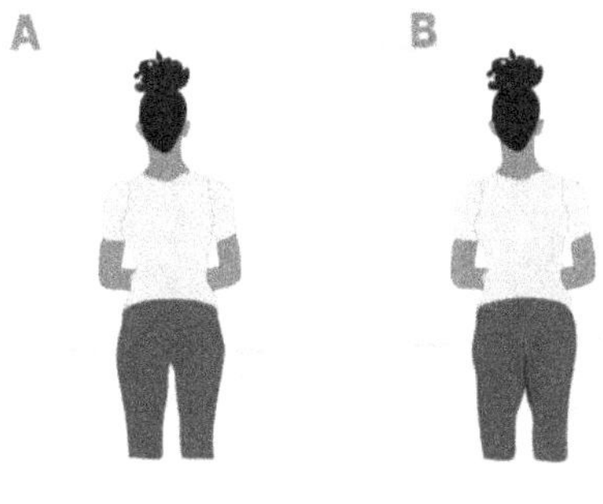

Butt squeezes

Ankle Pumps

1. Begin by lying on the floor on your back.

2. Elevate your legs by placing pillows or a short stool under your legs.

3. Flex your toes toward you, then point them away from you.

4. Repeat this movement 30 times.

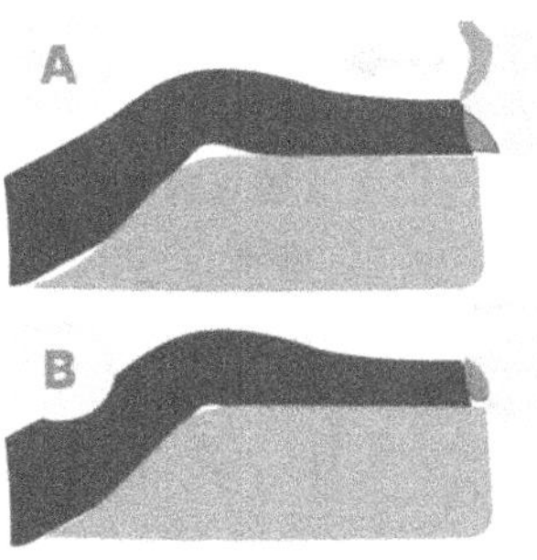

Ankle pumps

Heel to Toe Walk

1. For this exercise, begin by stepping your right foot forward in front of your left foot, going from heel to toe.

2. Your left toes should be touching your right heel.

3. Now place your left foot in front of your right foot with your right toes touching your left heel.

4. Keep walking forward like this for 20 steps, paying attention to moving from heel to toe.

5. Do three sets of 20 steps.

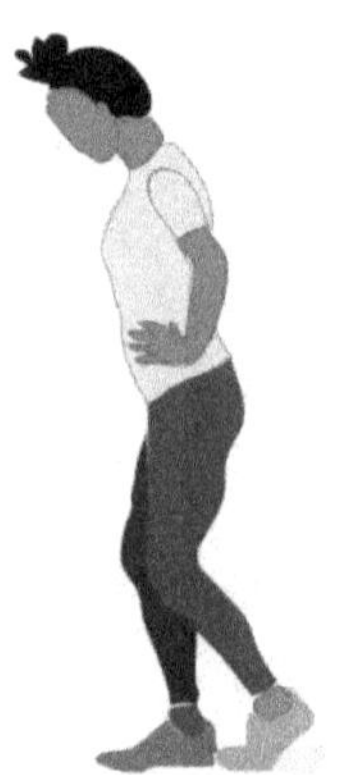

Heel to toe walk

Tightrope Walk

1. Stand with your feet together and your arms outstretched to your sides. Your arms should be parallel to the floor.

2. Begin walking in a straight line. This could be an imaginary straight line or you can draw a line on the floor.

3. Each time you lift your foot to step forward, hold it up for about two seconds, then release it slowly to the floor. Try to keep your body straight while doing this.

4. Complete 20 steps.

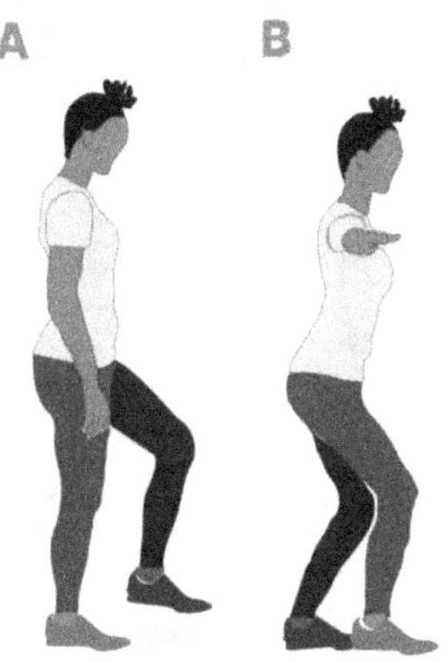

Tightrope walk

Rock the Boat

1. Stand with your feet shoulder-distance apart.

2. Extend your arms out to your sides to help with balance.

3. Look straight ahead as you slowly raise your right foot off the floor, lifting your leg.

4. Hold this position for about 30 seconds, then gently release your foot back to the floor.

5. Repeat this motion with your left leg.

6. Do this exercise five times on each side.

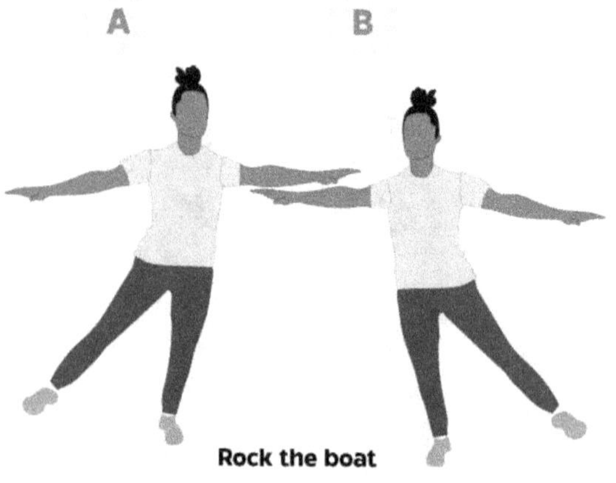

Rock the boat

Thigh Strengthening

Without the muscles in your thighs, you would not be able to stand up from sitting, walk up a flight of stairs, or maintain your balance. The muscles in our thighs are one of the areas affected as we age. If we do not work to maintain their strength, it becomes harder to perform day-to-day activities. This workout is geared to strengthening and toning your thigh muscles in order to help you maintain your self-sufficiency.

Sit to Stand

1. Begin by standing about six inches in front of a chair.

2. Lift your arms out in front of you for balance.

3. Slowly begin to bend your knees and sit back until your glutes touch the chair.

4. Hold here for a breath, then push up through your heels to come back to standing.

5. Repeat this move 8 to 12 times for two sets.

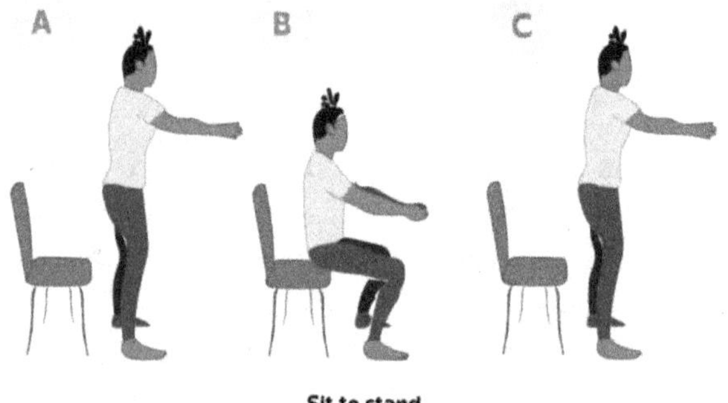

Sit to stand

Step Up

1. Stand in front of a step or low curb.

2. Step up with your right foot until your leg is straight, then step your left foot up.

3. Step down with your right foot, then your left foot.

4. Repeat this move ten times, switching legs halfway through. Do three sets.

5. You can add ankle weights for more of a challenge.

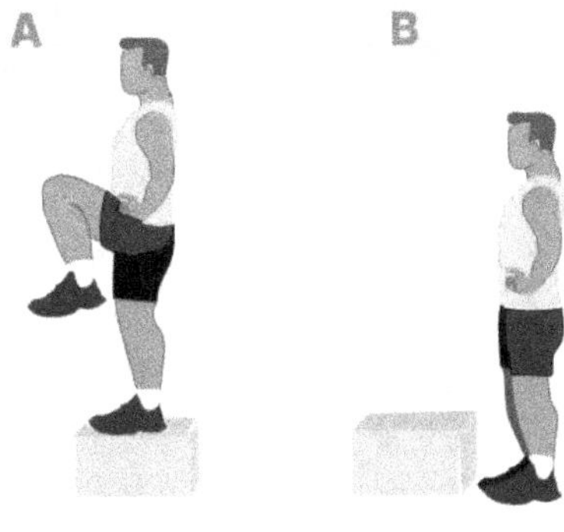

Step up

Single Leg Reach

1. Begin by standing with your feet hip-distance apart. You can do this exercise near a wall for additional support.

2. Extend both arms out to your sides at shoulder height.

3. Slowly lift your right foot about two inches off the floor.

4. Lean forward from your hips and touch your right hand to your left knee. Try not to round your back.

5. Pause here for a breath and then lift back up to your starting position without letting your right foot touch the floor.

6. Repeat this movement 8 to 12 times, then switch to the other side.

7. Complete two sets on each side.

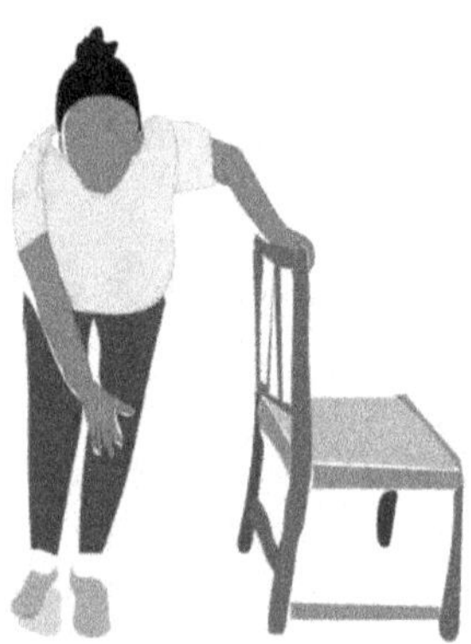

Single leg reach

Bridge

1. Start by lying on your back on the floor.

2. Place your feet flat on the floor with your knees pointing up toward the ceiling and your feet hip-distance apart.

3. Place your arms by your sides with your palms pressing into the floor.

4. Inhale and push through your heels, squeezing your glutes as you lift your hips up, creating a line from your knees to your shoulders.

5. Pause for a breath, then slowly, and with control, lower back down.

6. Complete two sets of 8 to 12 repetitions.

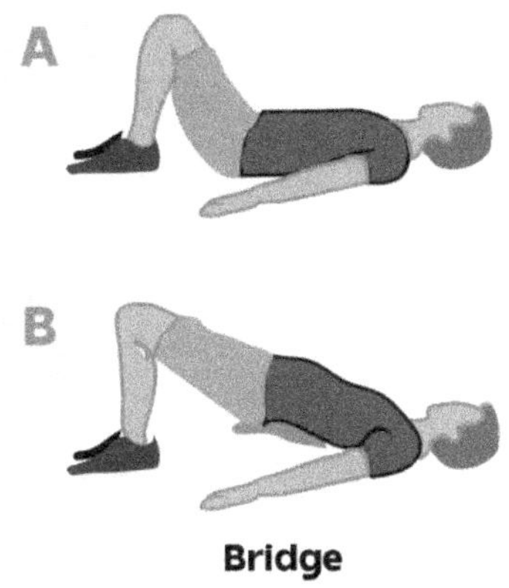

Bridge

Clamshell

1. Begin by lying on the floor on your right side with your knees bent and your legs stacked one on top of the other.

2. Keeping your feet together, slowly lift your left knee as far as feels comfortable, then lower it back down.

3. Repeat this movement 8 to 12 times for two sets, then switch to the other side.

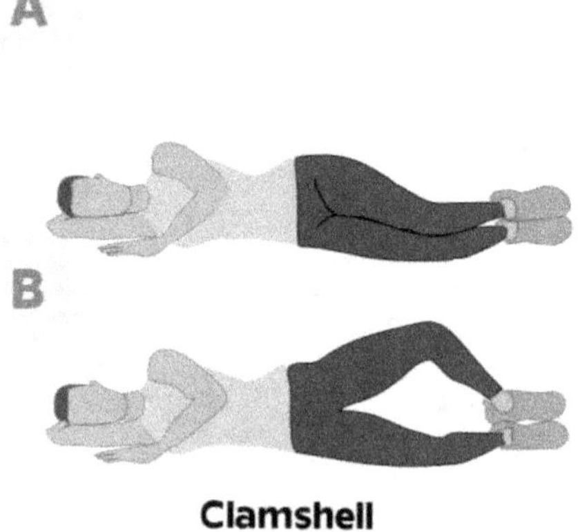

Clamshell

Wall Washer

1. For this exercise, it would be easier if you wore socks.

2. Lie on your right side with your back about six inches away from the wall.

3. Bend your right leg and keep your left leg straight.

4. Keeping your left leg straight, move it back until your left heel is pressing against the wall.

5. Now, slowly lift your leg, then lower it so it slides against the wall.

6. Do two sets of 8 to 12 repetitions on this side, then switch to the other side.

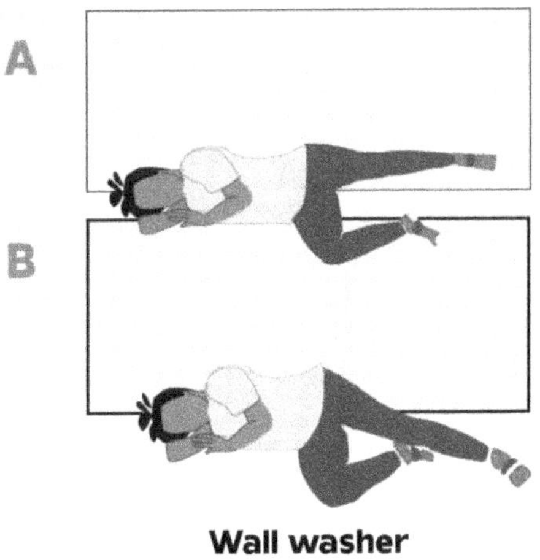

Wall washer

Calf Strengthening

Your calf muscles are essential for daily living and moving. Like the thigh muscles, they play a vital role in how you run, walk, and stand. Most of us have to work to develop, maintain, and strengthen our calf muscles, and this becomes even more vital as we age. The exercises in this routine will help you to build and strengthen these muscles.

Seated Calf Raises

1. Begin by sitting up tall in your chair with your feet flat on the floor, hip-distance apart.

2. Bring your feet back so that your heels are behind your knees.

3. Slowly raise your heels up off the floor as far as you can go, until you are on your toes.

4. Hold here for one breath, then slowly release your heels back to the floor.

5. Repeat this exercise ten times.

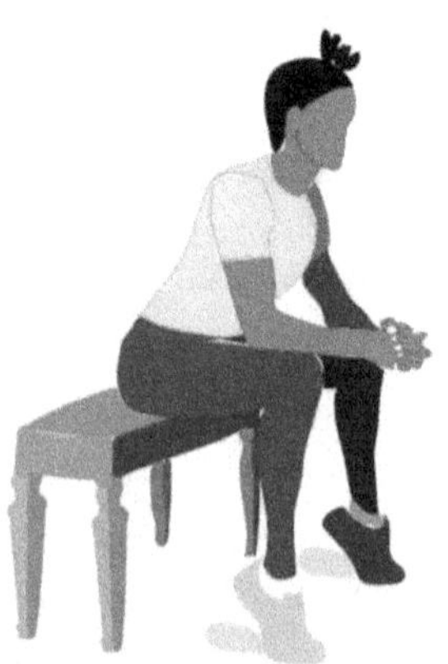

Seated calf raises

Standing Calf Raises

1. Stand behind a chair with your feet hip-distance apart.

2. Keep your knees straight and hold on to the back of the chair with both hands.

3. Slowly lift your heels up until you are standing on your toes.

4. Hold here for one breath, then gently release your heels back to the floor.

5. Repeat this movement ten times.

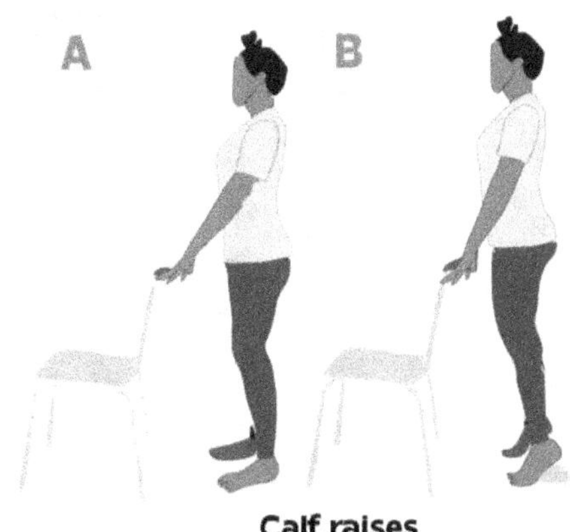

Calf raises

Elevated Calf Raises

1. Stand on a step or a workout stool with your feet hip-distance apart and your heels hanging off the edge.

2. Your weight should be balanced on the balls of your feet and your feet should be in line with your ankles. Use the stair rail or a wall for support and balance.

3. With control, lift your heels up to stand on your toes.

4. Hold for one breath, then slowly lower back to the starting position.

5. Repeat this move ten times.

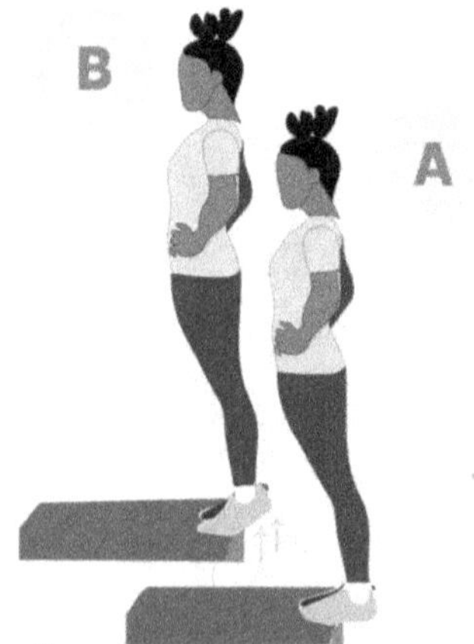

Elevated calf raises

Jump Rope

1. Stand in an area that has enough space around you for the rope to swing.

2. Begin with the rope behind you and hold the handles at hip level, slightly in front of your body.

3. Rotate the rope using a circular wrist motion. Keep your elbows at your sides and jump up without kicking your legs behind you.

4. Repeat this movement for about three to five minutes.

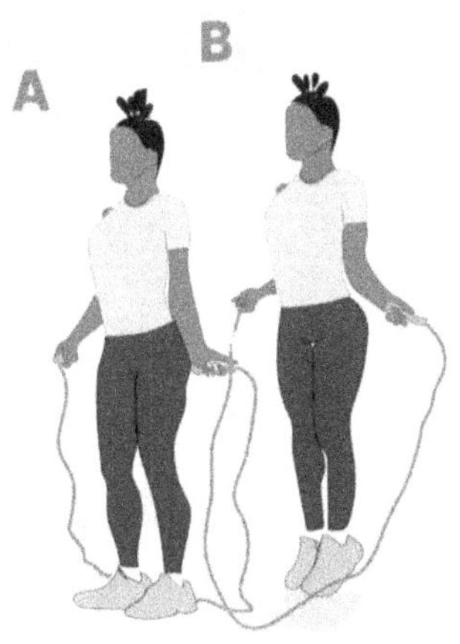

Jump rope

Single Leg Calf Raises

1. Stand behind a chair with your feet hip-width apart.

2. Use the back of the chair for support and lift your left foot off the floor slightly.

3. Slowly lift your right heel up until you are on your toes.

4. Hold here for one breath, then gently release your heel back to the floor.

5. Repeat this movement 1ten times with your right foot, then switch and repeat with your left foot, lifting your right foot slightly off the floor.

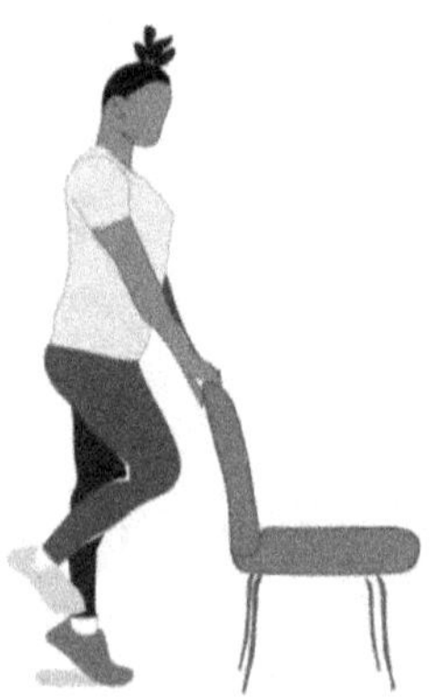

Single leg calf raise

Chapter 8:

Low Impact Cardio or Yoga

for Seniors

As we've already made clear, getting older shouldn't prevent you from moving. It might be more difficult if you have joint issues or other health-related ailments, but you can keep your joints and muscles mobile by doing low impact cardio or yoga.

Low impact exercises and yoga can offer all the benefits of a high-intensity workout without placing unnecessary stress on your joints and muscles. It can help to increase your strength, lower your blood pressure, and burn calories without causing pain. Yoga can also increase your balance and help to prevent falls.

Low Intensity Cardio Training

There is a common misconception that a workout can only be effective if it is intense, especially a cardio workout. This is a huge deterrent for many who cannot do high intensity training. Low intensity cardio training can provide the same benefits to your overall health in a more moderate and accessible way.

A low intensity cardio training is when you workout between 57 and 63% of your maximum heart rate for a continued period of time, usually about 30 minutes. This type of training can provide all the benefits of a high intensity session without placing stress on your joints. It can improve blood flow and circulation to the muscles, which is an important consideration as we age. The great advantage of low intensity cardio is that you can have a conversation while you work out, which makes it a fantastic exercise for socializing. Exercise is always better when you have company!

Incorporating low intensity cardio into your weekly routine can increase your body's ability to better use oxygen during exercise, which results in a better breakdown of carbohydrates and fats for energy. It also helps to transport oxygen more efficiently throughout your body.

Low intensity cardio training strengthens your heart, lungs, muscles, and bones, and reduces stiffness and pain in muscles and joints. It can also aid in the management of high blood pressure, diabetes, and heart disease. The best thing is that it is suitable for everyone at any fitness level.

Whether you prefer to get your exercise indoors or outdoors, there are a ton of different ways to get in a low intensity cardio workout. You can go for a walk or a hike, or use a treadmill. You can do exercises in the pool, swim laps, or even try a rowing machine if you don't feel like getting wet. If you want something a bit more fast-paced, you can try cycling or using an exercise bike. Any of these options, when committed to for 30 minutes, is an awesome way to get in a low intensity cardio workout without the stress.

Low Impact Cardio Workout

This can be done on its own or as a warm-up for a strength training workout. Each of these exercises should be done for one minute and can be adjusted to your fitness and mobility level. Remember to take a break when you need it.

Low Impact Jumping Jack

1. Begin by standing straight with your arms down at your sides.

2. Step your right foot out to the side and lift your arms above your head at the same time. Try to keep your weight on your right foot while doing this move.

3. Return to your standing position.

4. Now step your left foot out to the side, and again, lift your arms above your head. Make sure your weight is on your left foot.

5. Return to your first position and repeat this move on each side for one minute.

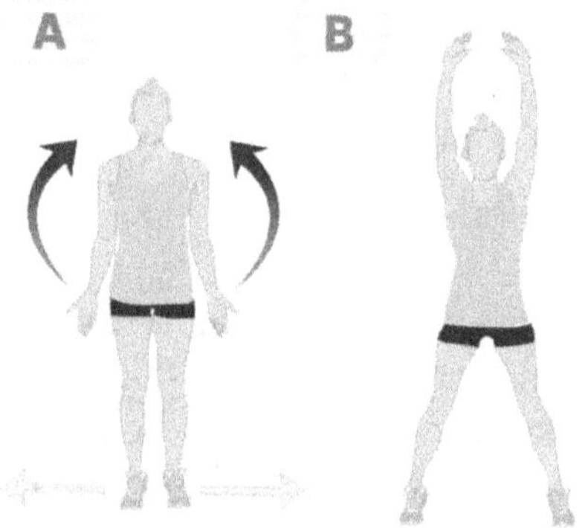

Low impact jumping jack

Skaters

1. Begin with your legs slightly wider than your shoulders and keep your arms at your sides.

2. Slightly bend your knees and bring your right leg behind and across your body. Lift your left arm up as you cross your right leg to give you stability.

3. Push off your left and begin to stand as you bring your right leg forward and cross your left leg behind you. Switch arms as you complete this movement.

4. Continue switching sides for one minute. Move as fast as you feel comfortable, but don't jump.

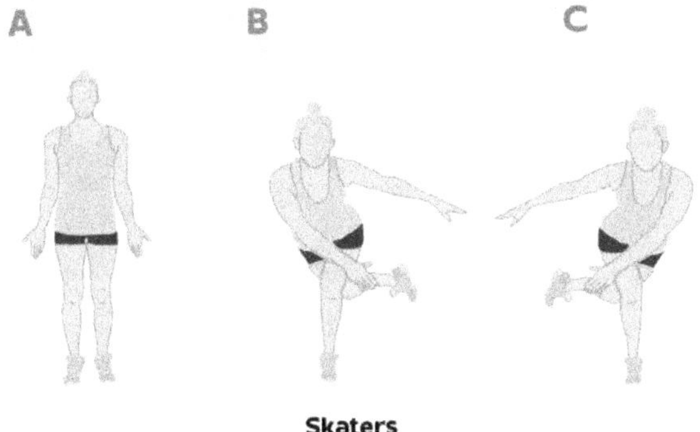

Skaters

Squat to Jab

1. Begin with your feet a bit wider than shoulder-distance apart and your arms at your sides.

2. Bend your knees in a squat, making sure to keep your chest up and your buttocks back, as if you're about to sit in a chair.

3. Raise up to a standing position, and throw a crossbody punch with each arm.

4. Return to your squat and lower your arms to your sides.

5. Repeat these movements for one minute.

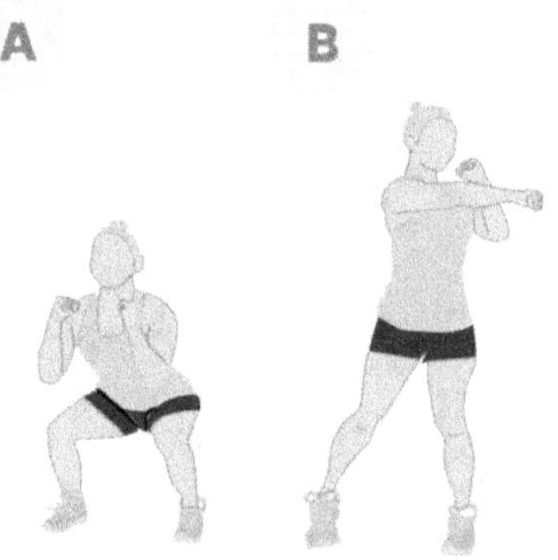

Squat to jab

Standing Oblique Crunch

1. Stand with your feet shoulder-distance apart and your hands behind your head with your elbows pointed out to either side.

2. Lean over to your right side as you bring your right knee up and your right elbow down, as if you want your right elbow to touch your right knee.

3. Lower your right leg and raise your right elbow, returning to your starting position.

4. Repeat this movement on your left side.

5. Continue to alternate this movement on your right and left sides for one minute.

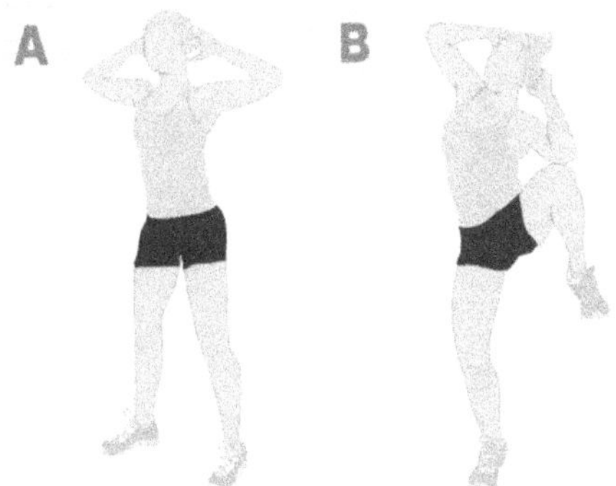

Standing oblique crunch

Lateral Shuffle

1. Begin with your feet shoulder-width apart and your knees slightly bent. Bend your elbows and lift your arms up close to your chest. Bend forward slightly.

2. Lift your right foot while pushing off with your left foot to move your body to the right. Try to do this as quickly as you can while maintaining your posture.

3. Bring your feet together and then repeat the shuffling movement to the right three more times.

4. Reverse your movements and shuffle four times to the left.

5. Keep shuffling equally in either direction for one minute.

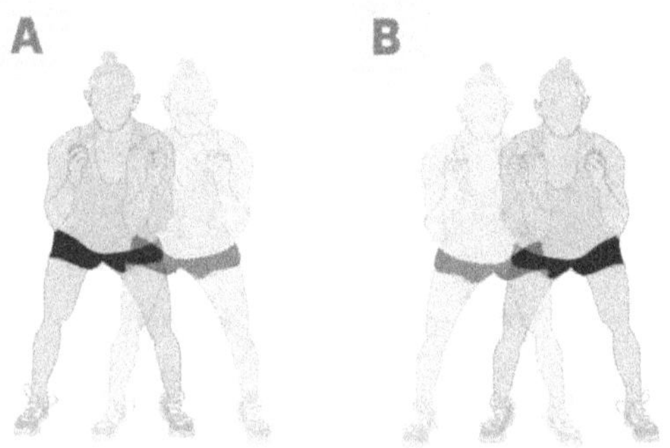

Lateral shuffle

Reverse Lunge Front Kick

1. Start with your feet shoulder-distance apart and your knees slightly bent. Bend your elbows and bring your arms up close to your chest.

2. Begin shifting your weight to your left leg as you kick your right leg out in front of you (it doesn't have to be a high kick). As you bring your right leg back down, step it back into a lunge.

3. Step back up into your starting position and repeat on the same side for 30 seconds.

4. After 30 seconds, switch to the other side and repeat with your left leg for another 30 seconds.

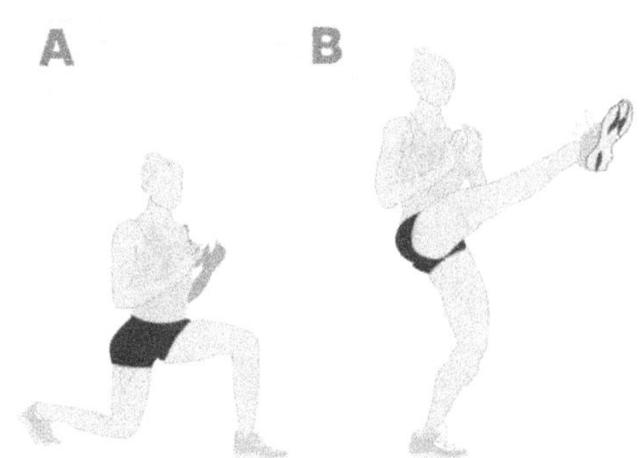

Reverse lunge front kick

Low Impact Cardio Yoga Sequence

Yoga is a great way to build strength, increase your flexibility, and improve your mobility without placing additional strain or stress on your joints and muscles. It can also help to improve your mood and reduce back pain.

1. Begin in a comfortable seated position with your spine nice and long, and your hands in prayer position.

2. Take your left hand to your right knee and your right fingers to your right shoulder. As you inhale, loop your shoulders back and draw your

right elbow gently up, over, and around, coming into an easy twist on your right. Exhale and slowly return to center.

3. Repeat this twist on your left side with your left hand on your left shoulder. Then return to the center.

4. Extend your arms out in front of you with your hands flexed up to the ceiling.

5. On an inhale, open your arms wide left to right pressing out to the sides. As you exhale, move your arms back to center. Repeat this three more times, moving with your breath.

6. Slowly move forward onto your hands and knees, coming into tabletop position. You can pad your knees to make it more comfortable if you need to. Check that your wrists are underneath your shoulders and your ankles are under your knees. Your knees should be hip-width apart. Make sure the tops of your feet are firmly pressing into your mat.

7. Press into the top of your left foot and curl your right toes under, extending your right leg back. Check that your chest and arms are not collapsing.

8. With your right leg extended, gently rock back and forth about five times, then return to tabletop position.

9. Open your knees as wide as your mat with your big toes touching. Send your hips back and down toward your heels, and stretch your hands out in front as you lower your chest and head to the ground in child's pose. Stay here for three breaths, then return to tabletop position.

10. Press into the top of your right foot and curl your left toes under, extending your left leg back. Again, check that your chest and arms are not collapsing.

11. With your left leg extended, gently rock back and forth about five times then return to tabletop position. Repeat child's pose for three breaths.

12. Return to tabletop position, then lift one foot forward, followed by the other, until you are in a forward fold. From there, slowly rise up to standing.

13. Clasp your hands behind you, bringing your shoulder blades together and opening your chest for a nice stretch. Stay here for three breaths, then release your arms to your sides.

14. On your next inhale, lift your arms forward and up with your fingertips reaching for the ceiling. As you exhale, bend your knees and open your arms out to the sides, gently twisting to the left. Inhale and rise back up to center.

15. As you exhale again, twist and open to your right. Repeat this twist two times on each side. When you return to center, gently lower your hands to prayer position at your heart.

16. From here, open your legs as wide as your mat, with your toes facing forward, while keeping a slight bend in your knees.

17. Turn your right toes out and turn your left toes slightly in. Inhale and open your arms out to the sides, coming to shoulder height.

18. On an exhale, slowly bend your right knee (to about a right angle), coming into Warrior II.

19. Inhale and straighten your right knee. Keeping your arms extended out, reach forward with your right hand bending at the waist. If you can, reach your right fingertips toward the ground, coming into triangle pose. On an exhale, lift back up.

20. Now, turn your right toes in and your left toes out. Exhale and slowly bend your left knee, coming into Warrior II on the other side.

21. Inhale and straighten your left knee. Keeping your arms extended out, reach forward with your left hand bending at the waist. If you can, take your left fingertips toward the ground, again coming into triangle pose. On an exhale, lift back up.

22. Keeping your legs wide, bring your hands to your waist. Exhale, drawing your elbows back and leaning forward with your chest first, coming into a wide-legged forward fold. Again, only go as far as feels good to you. Your hands may or may not touch the floor. Wherever you are, stay there for three breaths, then slowly come back up.

23. Bring your feet together and place your hands in prayer position. Bow your head and take three deep breaths to finish your practice.

Yoga for Balance

As we age, our bodies change. These changes can affect the way we walk, stand, and even sit. They can also affect our sense of balance. A regular yoga practice can help with your mobility, stability, and balance. These poses can be done in about 15 minutes every day to help you maintain movement and balance.

Mountain Pose

1. Stand up tall with your feet hip-width apart and your toes facing forward.

2. Keep your arms down by your sides with your palms facing forward and your fingers spread wide.

3. Roll your shoulders back and down, as if you are reaching your chest forward.

4. Try to place equal pressure on all four corners of your feet as you stand tall with your gaze forward.

5. Stay in this position for five breaths, focusing on your balance.

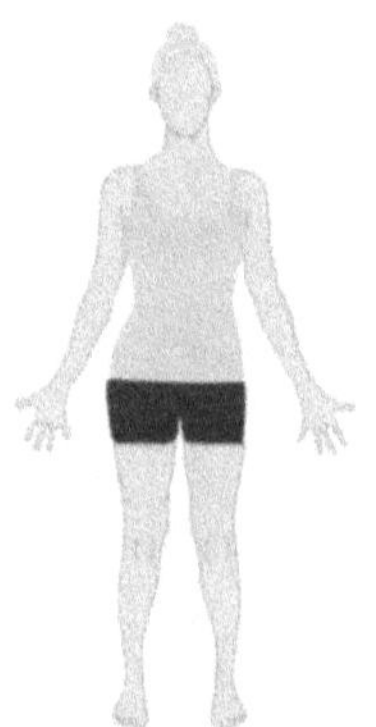

Mountain pose

Tree Pose

1. With your hands on your hips, stand with your feet hip-distance apart and your chest lifted.

2. Slowly shift your weight to your left foot and place the sole of your right foot on the inner ankle of your left foot, with your right knee pointing out to the right.

3. Try not to collapse into your left hip. Stay tall and firmly rooted through your left leg.

4. If you're comfortable, you can lift your hands into prayer position at your heart. Stay here for five breaths, then release back into your standing position.

5. Repeat this pose with your left leg and hold for another five breaths.

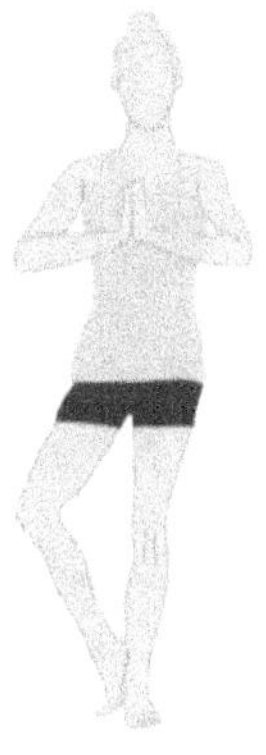

Tree pose

Warrior I

1. Begin in Mountain pose.

2. Slowly step your right foot back about three feet. Bend your left knee to a 90 degree angle and turn the toes of your right foot in, slightly toward your left leg.

3. Keeping your right left straight, slowly lift your arms up over your head toward the ceiling. Keep looking forward.

4. Hold this pose for five breaths, then return to Mountain pose.

5. Repeat these movements with your left leg.

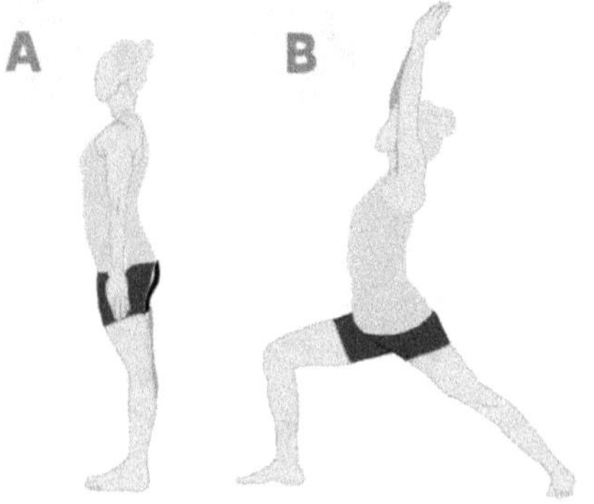

Warrior 1

One-Legged Mountain Pose

1. Begin in Mountain pose.

2. Slowly lift your left knee up to a point that feels comfortable. Don't go further than hip height. Keep your left foot flexed. You can also use a wall or chair to help with balance.

3. Hold this pose for five breaths, then release back to Mountain pose.

4. Repeat this with your right leg.

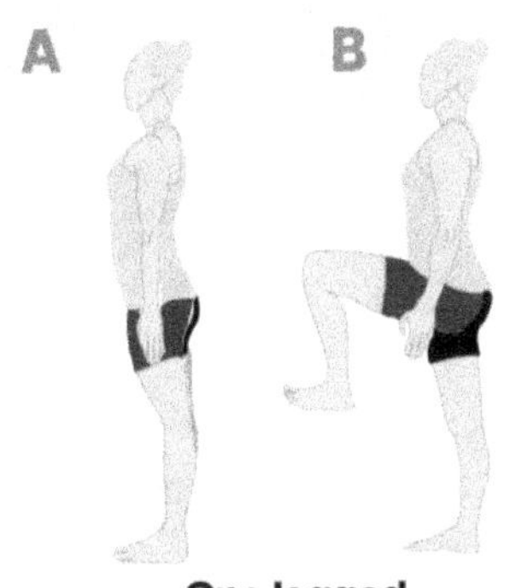

**One legged
mountain pose**

Modified Dancer's Pose

1. Start in Mountain pose.

2. Bend your right knee and bring your right foot back toward your buttocks.

3. Hold on to your right foot with your right hand while lifting your left hand up to the side of your face.

4. Press your right foot into your right hand as you hold this position for five breaths.

5. Release and return to Mountain pose.

6. Do this pose with your left leg.

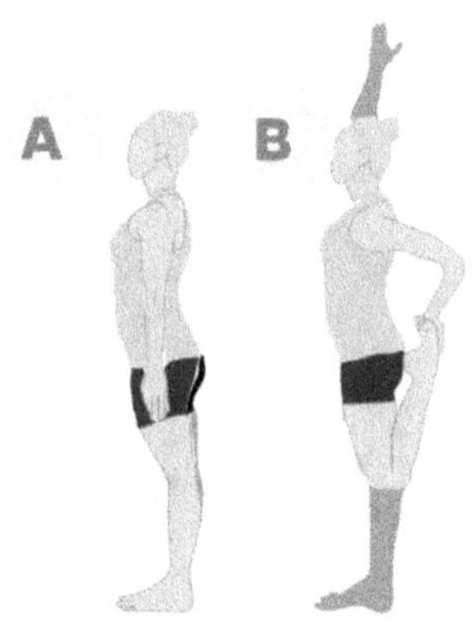

**Modified dancers
pose**

Chapter 9:

Core Strengthening

Exercises

When we talk about our core muscles, we are referring to the muscles in our abdomen as well as our back and along our spine, hips, and pelvis. Our core muscles support our lower back and help us to stand, lift, bend, get out of a chair, and balance. They also provide us with the stability we need to twist and turn. Basically, these muscles support the daily movements we often take for granted.

Like our other muscles, as we age, our core muscles can become weak from lack of use, as well as the aging process. If the muscles, tendons, and ligaments in your core are not strengthened regularly, the tissues become stiff and weak, leading to mobility issues. If we want to continue to live independently as we get older, then we need to ensure that we focus on strengthening the muscles of our core. More importantly, we need to do the right exercises that are beneficial and not harmful.

Let's start with the ones that can harm us: crunches and sit ups. These are probably the worst exercises that you can do, particularly as you get older. Sit ups and crunches only target and strengthen a few of the muscles that make up your core. In fact, these exercises train your hip flexors and not your core. If your hip flexors become too strong, they can pull on your lower back and result in back pain. Moreover, crunches and sit ups pose a serious risk for older adults because they can pull on your neck, causing pain and injury.

Instead of crunches and sit ups, opt for core routines that include bridges and planks (or modified planks). Doing bridge exercises actually contract all the muscle groups associated with the core without straining or pulling on any other muscles. Doing a proper plank strengthens not only your core, but your arms and shoulders as well. The trick is to stay as stiff as possible (just like a plank of wood).

When performing core exercises, focus on the quality of your movement rather than the quantity. If you're doing the move incorrectly or not engaging the right muscles, then no matter how many you do, it's not going to be as effective. Take your time and do it right. As you get stronger, you can add on more repetitions and more sets. The goal is to create a sustainable core routine.

A strong core can increase your overall body strength. Stronger muscles means that your range of motion improves which makes doing daily tasks easier and gives you a better reaction time. As you already know, your core muscles support your spine. So a stronger core boosts your balance, posture, and stability. This, in turn, provides a better center of gravity, giving you more confidence in your movements, therefore reducing your risk of falling and injury.

By stretching, lengthening, and toning the muscles of your core, you can better manage and even reduce chronic pain as well as symptoms of depression. Additionally, strengthening exercises can increase your bone density and help to maintain your existing muscle mass.

The routines in this section can be done individually or you can mix and match them to suit your needs or your fitness level. Always remember to complete a warm-up routine before you begin any strengthening exercises.

Low Impact Strengthening Exercises

Muscle loss is a natural path of aging, but that doesn't mean we can't prevent it or delay it. Doing a low impact strength training routine even once a week can make a difference to how you feel and move. It can also mean the difference between independence and reliance. This routine works toward overall strengthening of the body, and it may take time to build up to all the exercises, but the more regularly you do them, the easier they become.

Chin Up

1. When you stand or walk, try to keep your neck straight and your head up.

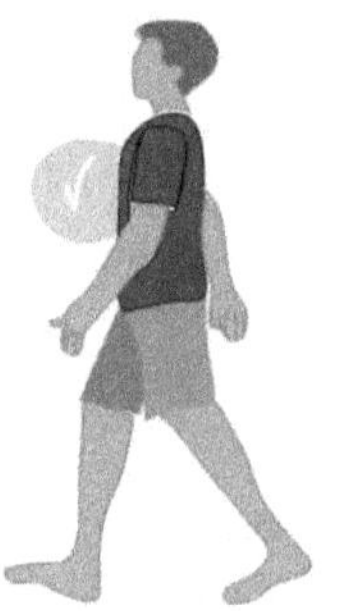

Chin up

Pec Stretches

1. Stand in the middle of a doorway with your feet hip-width apart.

2. Place your palms flat on either side of the doorway.

3. Gently step through, keeping your palms pressed to the doorway.

4. Hold for three breaths, then return to your starting position.

5. Repeat this movement five more times.

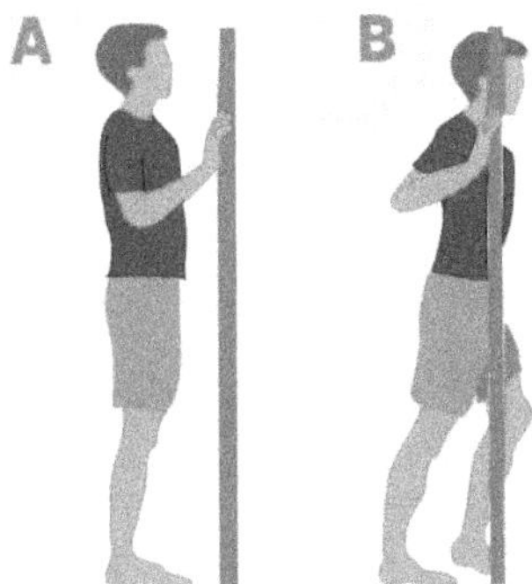

Pec stretches

Standing Balance

1. Begin by standing behind a chair or near a table with your feet shoulder-width apart.

2. Lift your right leg up and balance on your left foot. Use the chair or table for support.

3. Try to hold your balance for about a minute, then lower your right leg back to your starting position.

4. Switch to your left leg and repeat the movement.

5. As your balance gets better, you can try doing it with the chair or table for support.

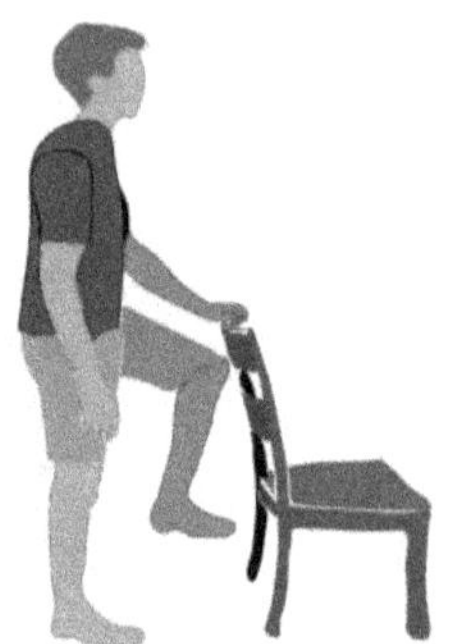

Standing balance

Lying Hip Bridges

1. Start by lying on your back with your knees bent and your feet flat on the floor. Your knees should be pointing up toward the ceiling.

2. Press your lower back into the floor, squeeze the muscles of your glutes, and push your hips up until you make a straight line from your knees to your shoulders.

3. Hold for a breath and slowly lower back down to the floor.

4. Repeat this move ten times.

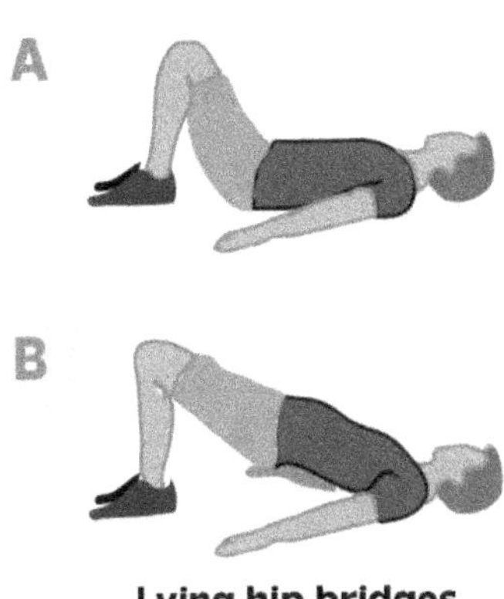

Lying hip bridges

Side Lying Circles

1. Begin by lying on your left side, keeping your body in a straight line and your legs stacked one on top of the other.

2. Extend your left arm straight up and rest your head on it.

3. Engage your core muscles and lift your right leg to about hip height (or as far as feels comfortable), then begin to make slow circles in a clockwise direction.

4. Do five circles in a clockwise motion, then reverse your circles and do five in a counterclockwise direction.

5. Slowly lower your right leg back to the start once you have completed circles in both directions.

6. Switch to the other side and repeat the same movements.

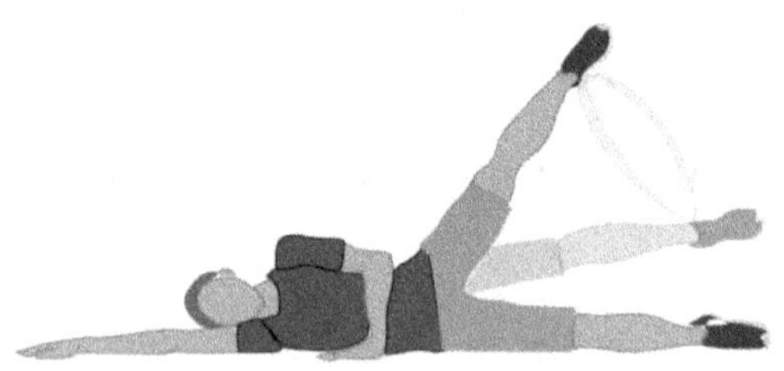

Side lying circles

Deadbugs

1. Begin by lying on your back with your hands and legs up in the air.

2. Bend your knees to a 90 degree angle so that your shins are parallel to the floor.

3. Keeping your lower back pressing into the floor, lower your right leg until your heel just touches the floor. At the same time, lower your left arm back over your head so that it touches the floor as well.

4. Lift your right arm back to the starting position.

5. Repeat this movement with your left leg and right arm.

6. Do this ten times on each side.

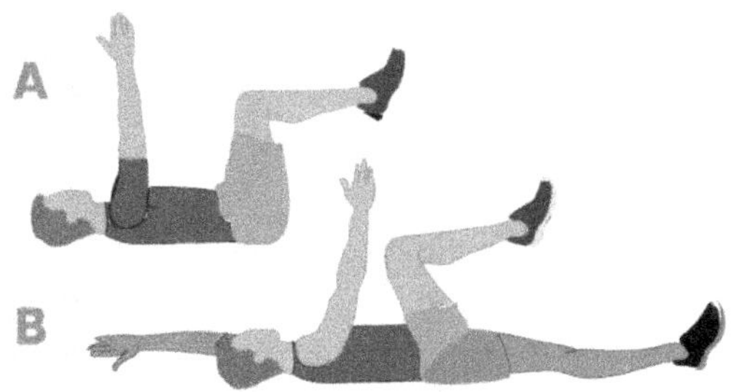

Deadbugs

Side Planks

1. Lie, propped up, on your left side with your left elbow directly under your shoulder and your legs extended in a straight line. Make sure that your legs are stacked one on top of the other.

2. As you engage your core muscles, lift your hips off the floor so that you create a straight line from your shoulders to your feet.

3. Hold here for five counts, then lower down to the floor.

4. Repeat this on the other side.

5. If having your legs extended is challenging, you can bend your knees, placing your feet behind you. Make sure to keep your knees stacked as you lift your hips up.

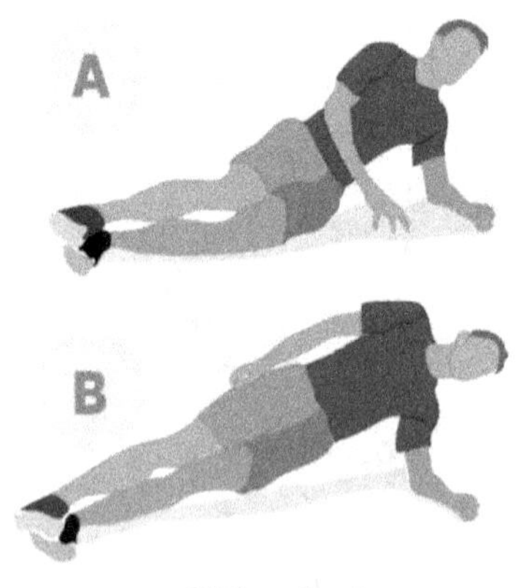

Side planks

Opposite Arms and Legs

1. Come to all fours on your mat, with your wrists directly under your shoulders and your knees under your hips.

2. Keep your back flat and your core muscles engaged.

3. Lift your right hand straight out in front of you as you extend your left leg out behind you.

4. Hold here for three breaths, then release back to all fours.

5. Repeat this exercise with your left hand and right leg.

6. Do this eight times on each side.

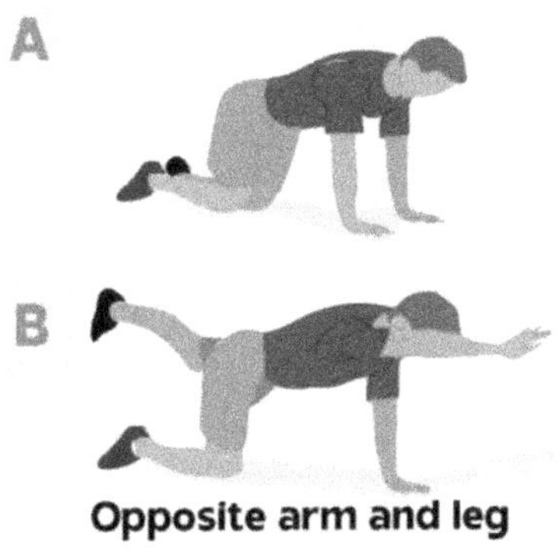

Opposite arm and leg

Squats With Chair Support

1. Stand in front of a chair with your feet hip-distance apart.

2. Lift your arms out in front of you to about shoulder height.

3. With your chest lifted and your back straight, slowly begin to push your hips back as you bend your knees, as if you were going to sit in the chair.

4. Just let your bum gently rest on the chair as you lower down. Your upper body should only be leaning slightly forward.

5. Pause in your squat for one breath.

6. To lift back up, push firmly and evenly into your feet, squeezing your glutes as you return to standing.

7. Repeat this movement eight times.

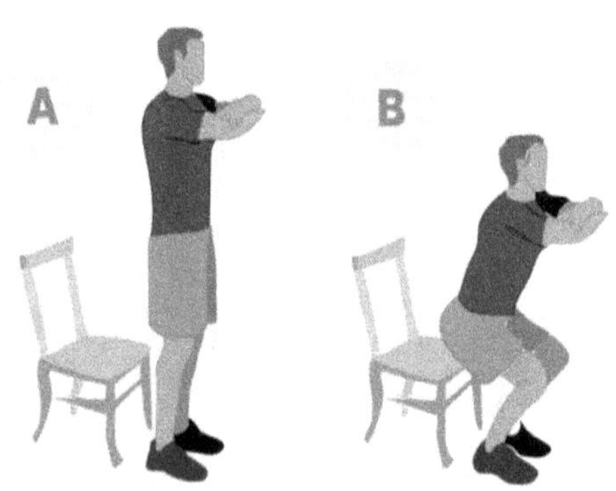

Squats with chair support

Wall Slides

1. Stand about one to two feet away from the wall with your feet hip-width apart and your toes pointing forward.

2. Lean back until your head, shoulders, arms, back, and buttocks are against the wall.

3. Slowly begin to lower your body by bending your knees until you get to about a 90 degree angle (or as far as feels comfortable for you).

4. Hold here for three breaths, then gently rise back up to your starting position.

5. Repeat this motion ten times for two sets.

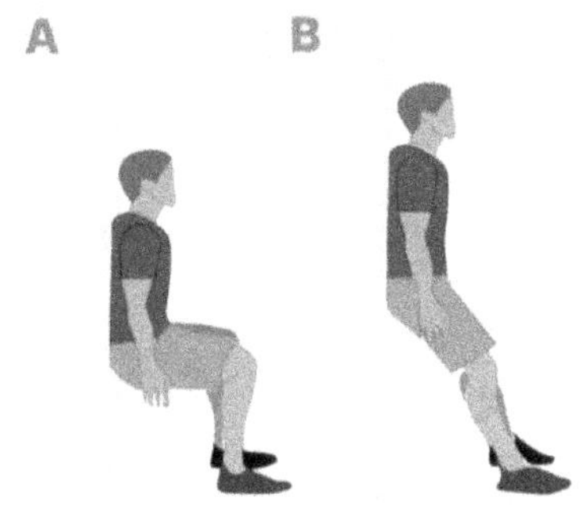

Wall slides

Wall Angels

1. Begin by standing with your back against the wall and your heels about three to six inches away from the wall.

2. Keep your feet hip-width apart and your arms down at your sides. The back of your head should be touching the wall. Tuck your chin to your chest.

3. Turn your palms to face out and slowly lift your arms up, keeping them against the wall.

4. Lift your arms as high as they can go without having to bend your elbows or feel any pain.

5. Hold here for a breath, then lower back down to your starting position.

6. Do this move about ten times.

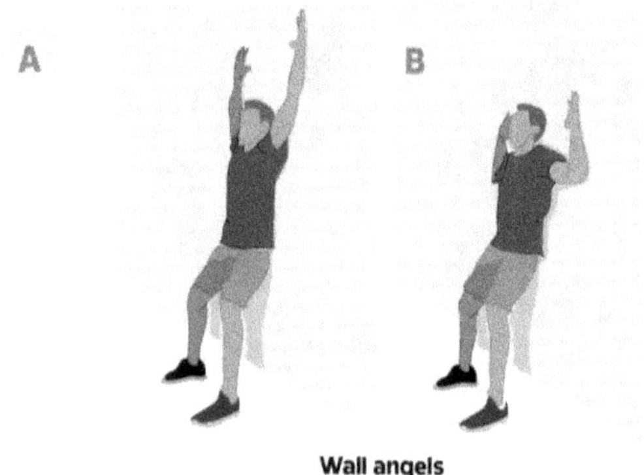

Wall angels

Wall Push-Ups

1. Stand about two feet away from the wall (closer if you need to make it easier) with your feet hip-width apart.

2. Place your palms flat on the wall with your fingers spread wide. Your hands should be at shoulder height and shoulder-distance apart.

3. Slowly bend your elbows out to your sides to lower your chest to the wall. Allow your heels

to lift up off the floor. Be sure to keep your body in a straight line.

4. Hold for one breath, then press firmly through your palms to rise back up to your starting position.

5. Repeat this ten times. As you get stronger, you can add more sets.

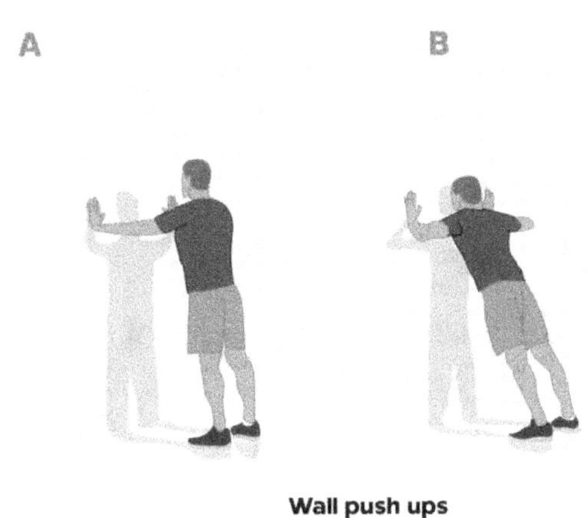

Wall push ups

Back Strengthening

As we get older, on many occasions we tend to move less, and this can contribute significantly to back pain and discomfort. The more we move, the better it is for our muscles and our general health. Strengthening our back means we can move easier and more confidently, and our reaction time will be better.

Cat Cow

1. Begin on all fours with your wrists directly under your shoulders and your knees under your hips.

2. Keep your back straight and your neck long.

3. As you inhale, lift your head up and arch your back, coming into a 'U' shape.

4. On your exhale, lower your head, round your back, and look at your belly.

5. Repeat this cycle eight times. Do three sets.

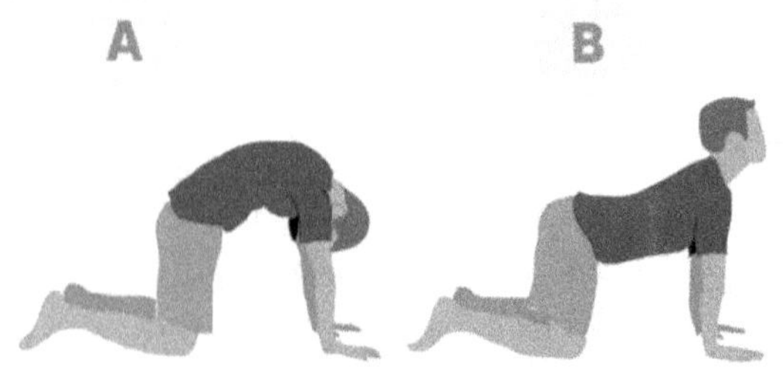

Cat cow

Glute Bridge

1. Begin by lying on your back with your knees bent and the soles of your feet flat on the floor. Your knees should be pointing toward the ceiling.

2. Keep your feet and knees hip-width apart. Rest your arms down along the side of your body with your palms facing down.

3. Engaging the muscles of your core, lift your hips and pelvis off the floor, as far as feels comfortable.

4. Hold here for one breath, then slowly release back to the floor.

5. Repeat this movement 10 to 12 times.

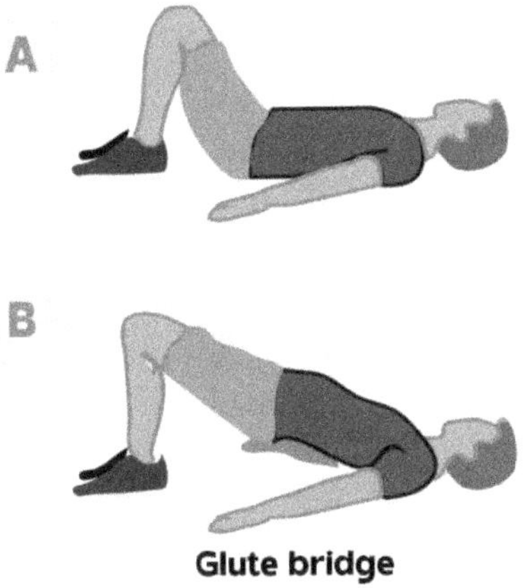

Glute bridge

Arm Raises

1. Lie on your back with your legs extended and your arms down at your sides.

2. As you inhale, slowly lift your right arm up until your fingers are pointing up toward the ceiling. If this feels uncomfortable, only lift your arm as far as feels good to you.

3. Exhale and gently lower your right arm back down to your side.

4. On your next inhale, lift your left arm, then lower it on an exhale.

5. Repeat this movement eight times for three sets.

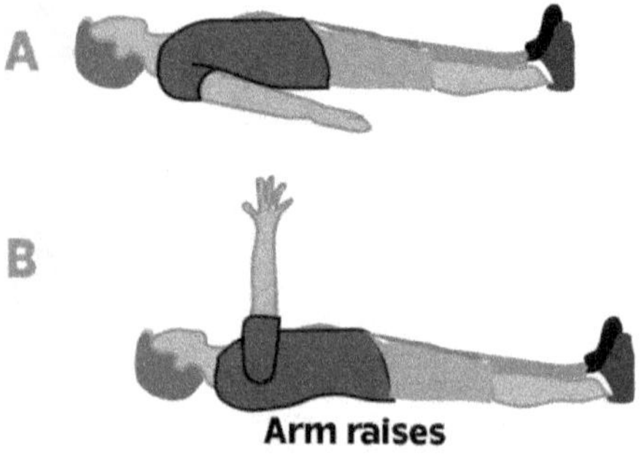

Arm raises

Knee Hugs

1. Lie on the floor with your legs extended and your arms resting down at your sides. For added support, you can place a pillow under your lower back.

2. Bend your right leg and bring your knee up toward your chest, or as close as you can get it.

3. Wrap your arms around your right knee and hug it into your chest. Hold here for about five seconds, then lower your right leg back to the floor.

4. Repeat with your left leg.

5. Do this eight times with each leg. You can also try to hug both knees at the same time for a deeper stretch.

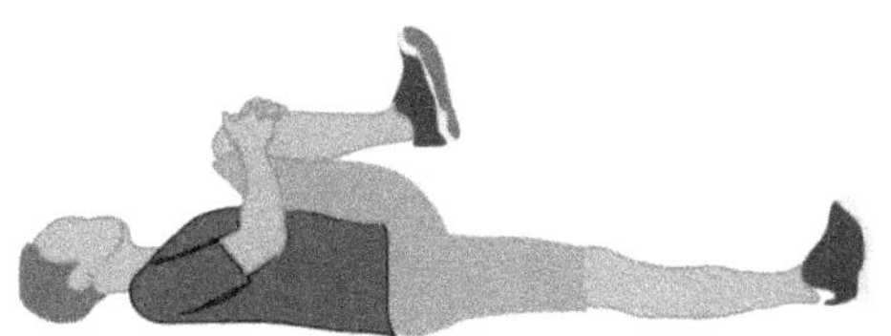

Knee hugs

Seated Neck and Chest Stretch

1. Sit in a comfortable chair with your feet flat on the floor, hip-width apart.

2. Interlace your finger behind your head so that your elbows are pointing out to the sides like triangles. You can leave your thumbs resting on the sides of your neck for extra support.

3. Gently lift your chin up, tilting your head back slightly, and opening your chest.

4. Inhale deeply.

5. On your exhale, bend toward your right so that your right elbow is slightly angled toward the floor.

6. On your inhale, return to your starting position.

7. Exhale and bend to your left side, angling your left elbow toward the floor. Inhale and return to center.

8. Repeat this movement five times for three sets.

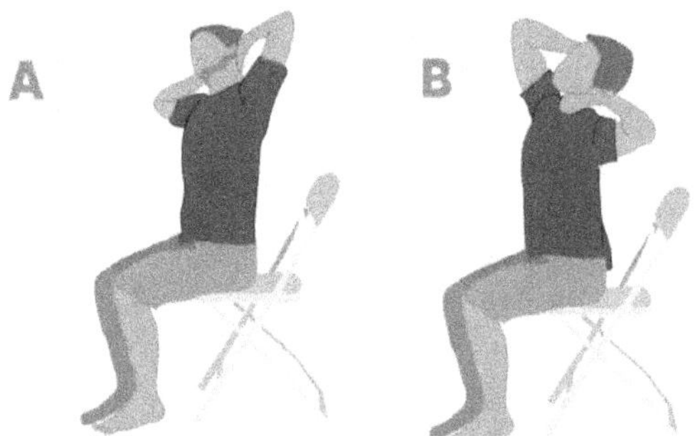

Seated neck and chest stretch

Shoulder Shrugs

1. Sit up tall in a comfortable chair with your feet flat on the floor.

2. Inhale and lift your shoulders up toward your ears.

3. As you exhale, lower your shoulders back to your neutral position, away from your ears.

4. Repeat this motion five times.

5. For more of a challenge, you can hold small weights in both hands.

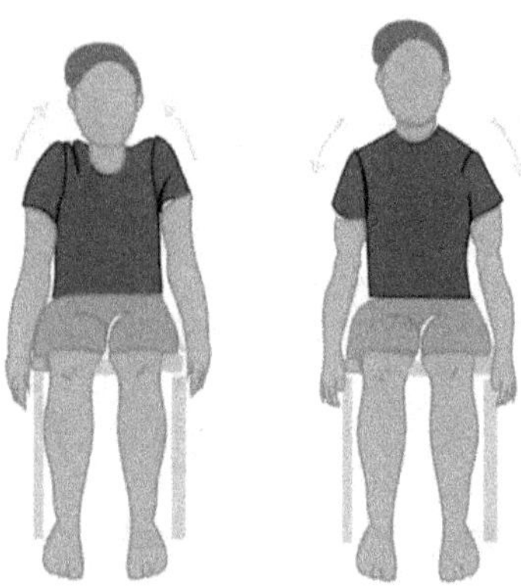

Shoulder shrugs

Hip Hinges

1. Begin by standing tall with your feet shoulder-distance apart.

2. With your hands on your hips and your core engaged, bend your knees slightly and begin to lean forward from your hips, keeping your back straight.

3. Depending on your range of motion, you can release your hands to the floor for a deeper stretch, but this isn't necessary.

4. Press firmly into your feet, and keeping your back straight, lift back up from your hips.

5. Repeat this exercise ten times.

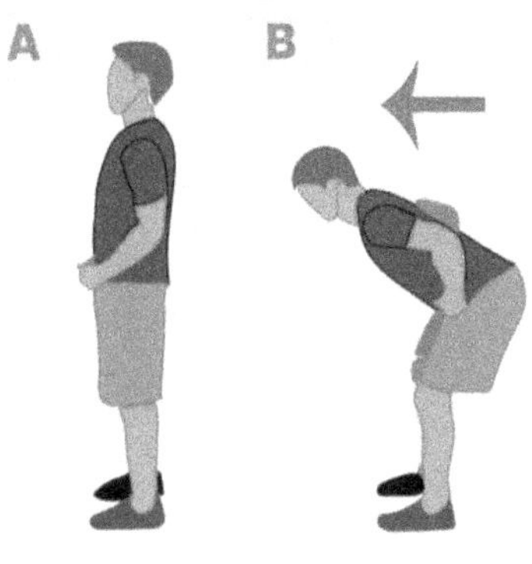

Hip hinges

Lumbar Extension

1. Stand with your feet hip-width apart and facing forward. Rest your hands on your hips for balance.

2. Gently begin to bend up and back as if you're bending over a ball. Only go as far as feels comfortable for you.

3. Stay in this bend for two breaths, then release back to your standing position.

4. Repeat this bend 8 to 12 times.

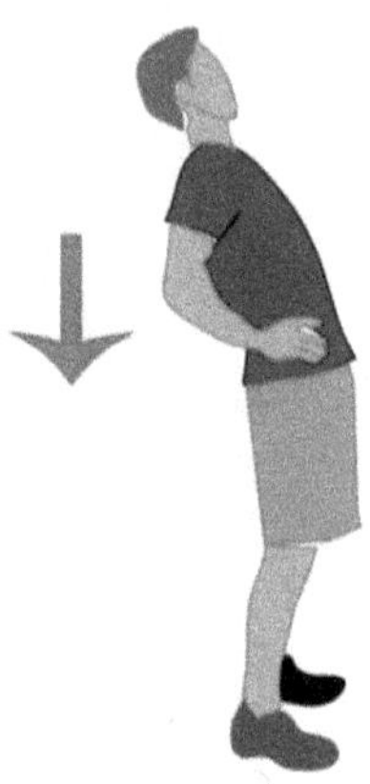

Lumbar extension

Leg Lifts

1. Start by standing behind a chair with your feet hip-width apart.

2. Hold on to the back of the chair with both hands for support.

3. Slowly lift your right leg slightly off the ground and out behind you.

4. Hold here for five seconds, then release.

5. Switch to your left leg and do the same movement.

6. Do this exercise five times on each side for three to five sets.

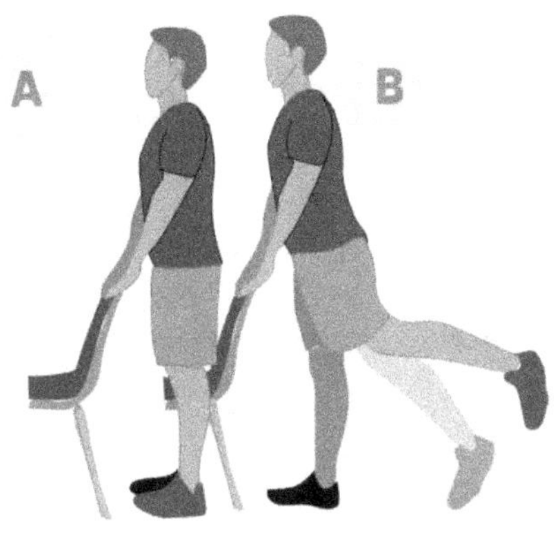

Leg lifts

Bird Dog

1. Come to all fours with your wrists under your shoulders and your knees under your hips.

2. Lift your left leg up and extend it out behind you.

3. Once you have your balance, reach your right arm straight out in front of you.

4. Hold here for five seconds, then return your arm and leg back to your starting position.

5. Repeat this movement with the other arm and leg.

6. Try to do this exercise ten times.

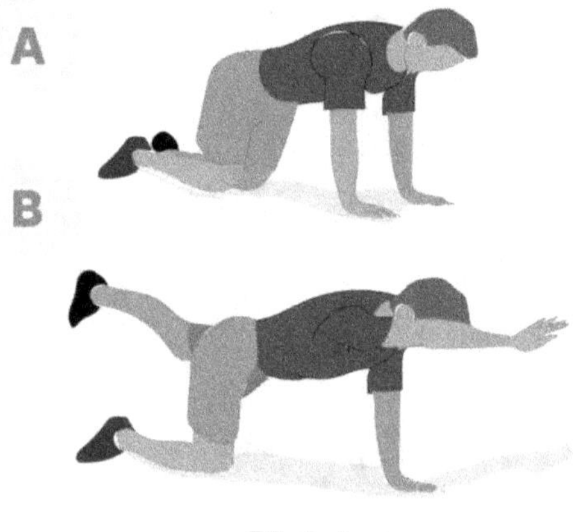

Bird dog

Core Strength

Core exercises improve your coordination, stamina, and stability, and aid in injury prevention. They also help you to manage and reduce pain, making your daily tasks easier. With a better center of gravity, you will be more confident in your movements and decrease your chances of falling.

Abdominal Crunch

1. Begin by lying on your back.

2. Place the soles of your feet flat on the wall so that your knees are at a 90 degree angle, and cross your hands over your chest.

3. Engage your core muscles and lift your head
    and shoulders off the floor.

4. Hold here for three breaths, then lower back to
    the floor.

5. Repeat this movement four times.

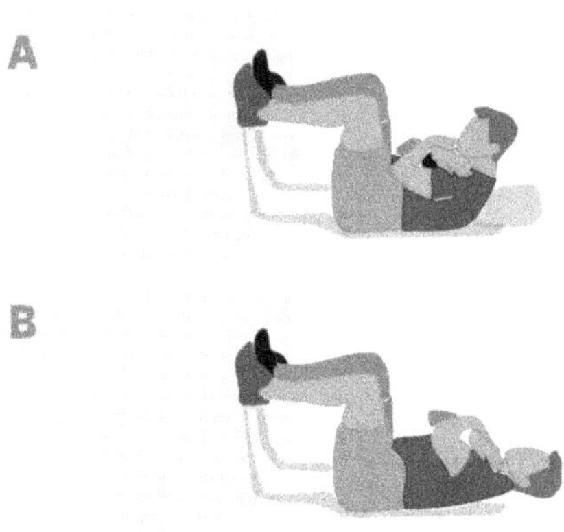

Abdominal crunch

Bridge

1. Begin by lying flat on your back with your spine
    in a neutral position. Bend your knees and place
    your feet flat on the floor. Rest your arms out
    to the sides.

2. Lift your hips off the floor as far as you can go
    and hold here for three breaths.

3. Slowly release your hips back to the floor.

4. Repeat this motion three to four times.

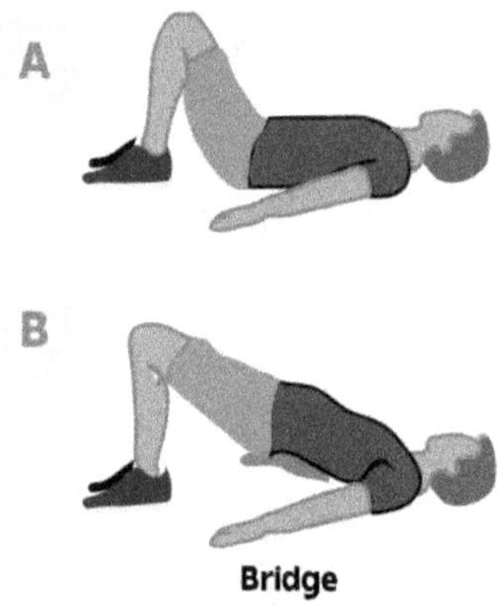

Bridge

Single Leg Ab Press

1. Lie on your back with your feet flat on the floor, hip-width apart, and your knees pointing up to the ceiling. Try not to tilt your hips.

2. Lift your right leg off the floor so that your knee is bent at a 90 degree angle and your shin is parallel to the floor.

3. Touch your right hand to your right knee.

4. Push your right hand against your knee and push your knee into your right hand at the same time. Keep your arm straight.

5. Hold here for three breaths, applying equal pressure, then return to your starting position.

6. Switch to your left leg and left hand.

7. Do this move three to four times on each side.

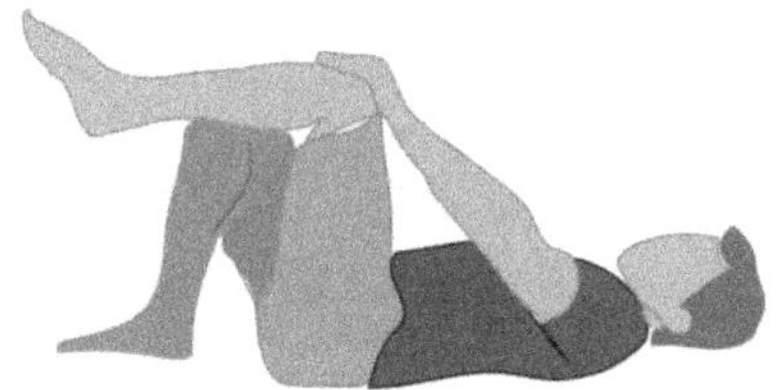

Single leg ab press

Double Leg Ab Press

1. Start by lying on your back with your knees bent and your feet flat on the floor.

2. Engage your core muscles and lift your legs off the floor, one at a time, so that your knees are bent at a right angle and your shins are parallel to the floor.

3. Place both your hands on your knees.

4. Pull your knees toward your chest as you push your hands against your knees.

5. Hold here for three breaths, then gently release back to your starting position.

6. Repeat this exercise three to four times.

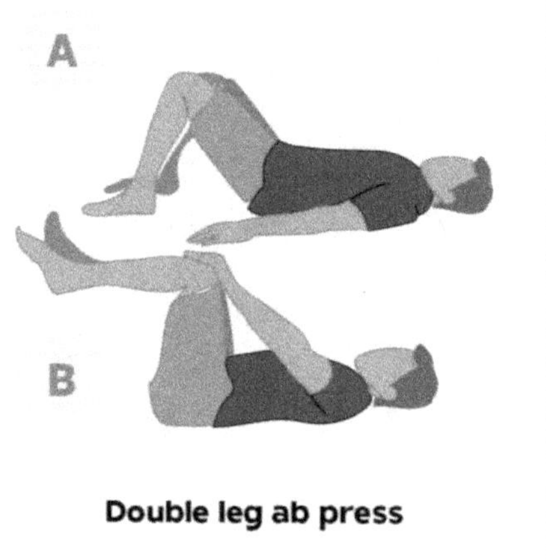

Double leg ab press

Spinal Twist

1. Lie on your back with your feet flat on the floor and your knees pointing up to the ceiling. Your feet and knees should be hip-width apart.

2. Keep your arms gently resting at your sides.

3. Slowly let your knees fall to the left while keeping your upper body steady. Only go as far as you can without feeling any discomfort. You should feel a stretch, but it should not be uncomfortable.

4. Stay in this twist on your left side for three breaths, then return to your starting position.

5. Now, repeat the twist on your right side.

6. Complete this spinal twist three to four times on each side.

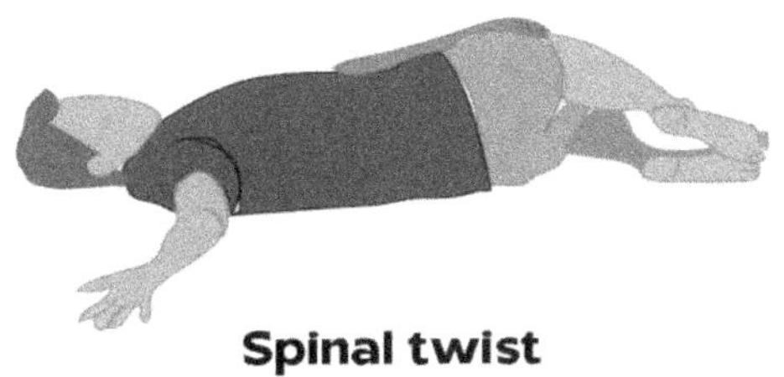

Spinal twist

Quadruped

1. Begin on all fours. Check your alignment to ensure that your knees are under your hips and your wrists are under your shoulders, as well as that your weight is equally distributed on your hands and knees.

2. Lift your left arm up and straight out in front of you. Hold for three breaths, then return your hand back to the floor.

3. Now lift your right arm up and straight out in front of you. Stay here for three breaths, then lower your right arm back to the start.

4. Lift your left leg up and extend it out behind you as high as feels comfortable (but no higher than your hip). Hold here for three breaths, then release your left leg back to the ground.

5. Repeat the same with your right leg.

6. Complete this cycle of movement three to four times.

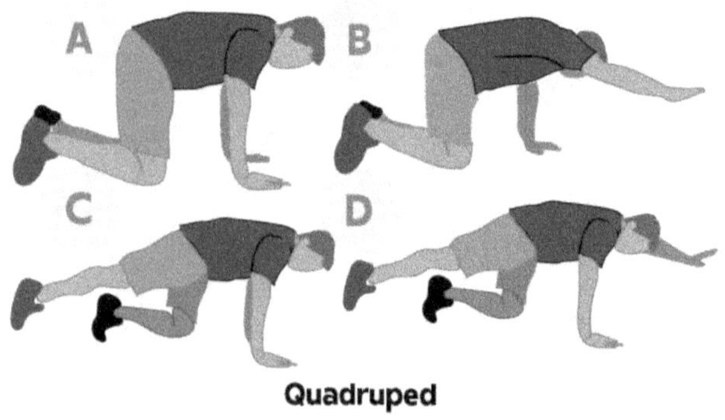

Quadruped

Side Plank

1. Lie on your right side, lifting yourself up onto your right elbow and forearm. Extend your legs out and stack them one on the other. Keep your left arm along the side of your body.

2. Slowly lift your hips off the floor as far as feels comfortable.

3. Hold for three breaths, then slowly lower back down.

4. Do this movement three to four times on this side, then switch to your left side and repeat.

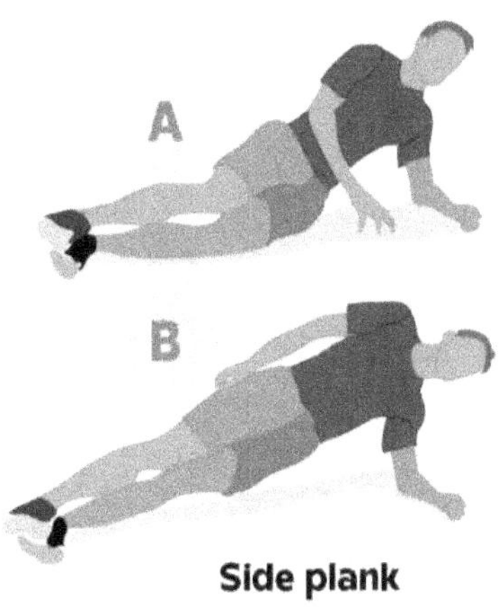

Side plank

Superman

1. Lie on your stomach with a pillow under your hips for support and a rolled towel under your forehead.

2. Extend your legs out behind you and your arms in front of you.

3. Slowly lift your right arm up and hold for three breaths, then lower back down.

4. Repeat with your left arm.

5. Now lift your right leg up and hold for three breaths, then release.

6. Switch to your left leg and repeat.

7. Repeat this exercise three to four times on each arm and leg.

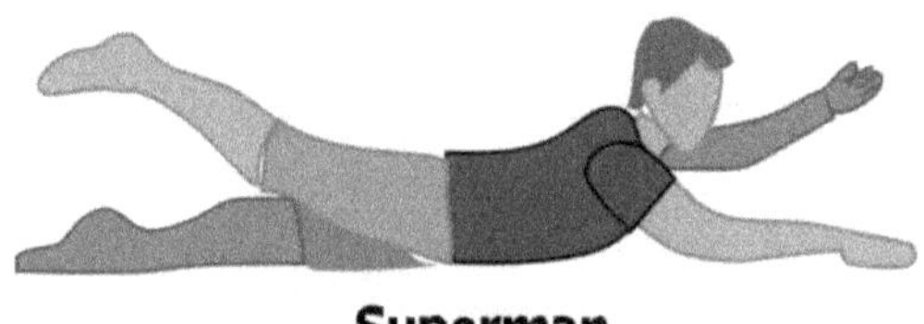

Superman

Chapter 10:

Chair Yoga for Strength and Mobility

In recent times, yoga has gained increasing popularity, especially in the West. Yoga is, in fact, an integral part of ancient Eastern traditions, and has been practiced for centuries. It blends movement with breathing in a manner that encourages mental, physical, and emotional well-being. Yoga comes in many different forms and practices, but they all have the same end goal: mind, body, and spirit wellness.

For many of us, particularly as we age and become less confident in our movements, yoga can seem daunting and out of our reach. Don't worry: Chair yoga can make a difference. It provides all the benefits of a traditional yoga practice while keeping you firmly grounded in a chair. A regular yoga practice can help with pain and stress relief, as well as joint lubrication and balance. It will also build strength in your arms, legs, and core, meaning you will be able to stand, sit, walk, and get up with ease.

We already know that as we get older, our muscles weaken. This weakening occurs especially in our legs, hips, and core, with the functioning of our brain changing and declining as well. All of these changes can lead to pain and discomfort in performing daily tasks, as well as impaired memory. Chair yoga can work to improve and maintain our spine health and even slow down some of the effects of aging. It can also halt the deterioration of our brain function.

As I've discussed at length, as older adults, one of our main causes of worry and anxiety is the loss of our independence and self-sufficiency. The stress caused by this can be overwhelming. Practicing yoga can help to soothe your mind, as well as your body, therefore lowering the body's stress response. By practicing yoga often, in a peaceful environment, you can alleviate your stress and find tranquility.

This chapter has been carefully created to focus on seniors who would like to begin or continue a yoga practice. It provides step-by-step instructions for a variety of poses, as well as variations depending on your comfort level. You can practice the sequence as a stand alone, or you can do it in conjunction with other exercises for a longer practice.

The poses detailed here are a great foundation on which to build your practice. They will help you to focus on your breathing while engaging your muscles. You will find yourself paying more attention to your posture and how you move, while increasing the mobility in your joints and hips, as well as the flexibility in your legs and arms. These yoga poses will help you stretch, lengthen, and strengthen the muscles in your upper and lower body, while teaching you how to release tension in your shoulders, jaw, and face. The end result will be a more confident and stronger you, capable of completing daily tasks with ease.

Chair Yoga Sequence

Seated Mountain Pose

1. Inhale and sit up tall in an armless chair. Imagine that you are being pulled up by a string and your spine is being lifted up.

2. Focus on keeping your feet flat on the floor and your knees hip-width apart with your toes pointing forward. Place your hands gently on your thighs with the palms facing down.

3. Breath in deeply, and as you exhale, gently roll your shoulders back and down away from your ears.

4. Use the muscles of your core to keep yourself sitting up tall, and at the same time, press down into the seat of your chair, letting your sitting bones become heavy. Keep your feet firmly pressed into the floor.

5. Stay here for five slow, deep breaths.

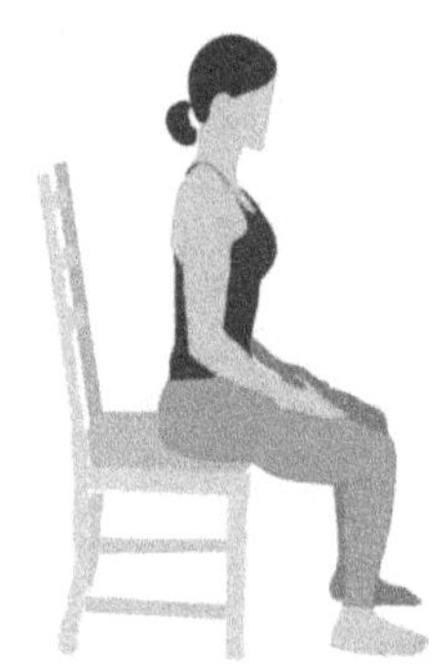

Seated mountain pose

Seated One-Legged Mountain Pose

1. Starting in Mountain pose, sit up tall with your feet pressed into the floor and your shoulders relaxed, down away from your ears. Your knees should be bent at 90-degree angles to the floor.

2. As you breathe in, slowly lift your right knee up, pause for one breath, and then lower it on an exhale. Only lift your knee as high as it feels comfortable. There should not be any pain or discomfort.

3. Do this five times with each leg, focusing on your breathing, then return to Mountain pose.

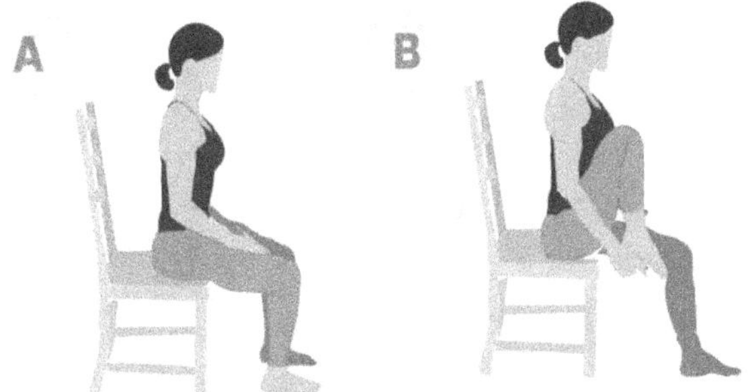

One legged mountain pose

Side Neck Stretches

1. Start by coming into Mountain pose.

2. As you breathe in, extend your spine and sit up as tall as you can.

3. Exhale and slowly tilt your right ear toward your right shoulder, lengthening through the left side of your neck. Notice if you are holding any tension in your shoulders and try to relax them away from your ears by rolling them back and down. Stay here for two breaths.

4. On your next inhale, lift your head back up to a neutral position.

5. Exhaling again, tilt your left ear to your left shoulder. Again, pay attention to where your shoulders are and try to keep them relaxed and down, away from the ears.

6. Breathe in and return your head to its neutral position.

7. Try to do this pose at least three times on each side. Do as many as feels comfortable to you, or as many as you feel your body needs.

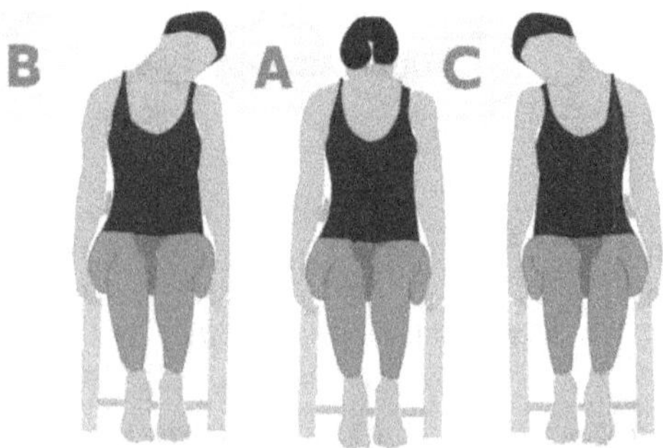

Side neck stretches

Shoulder Rolls

1. Begin in Mountain pose with your spine straight and your shoulders relaxed away from your ears.

2. As you inhale, lift your shoulders up, then back.

3. On your exhale, bring your shoulders down and around back to your starting position. You should make a full circle with your shoulders with each cycle of breath.

4. Keep the movement of your shoulders smooth and steady.

5. After five circles in this direction, reverse the movement, bringing your shoulders up and forward as you inhale, and down and around as you exhale. It may feel slightly odd moving in this direction, but that's normal. Complete five circles in this direction.

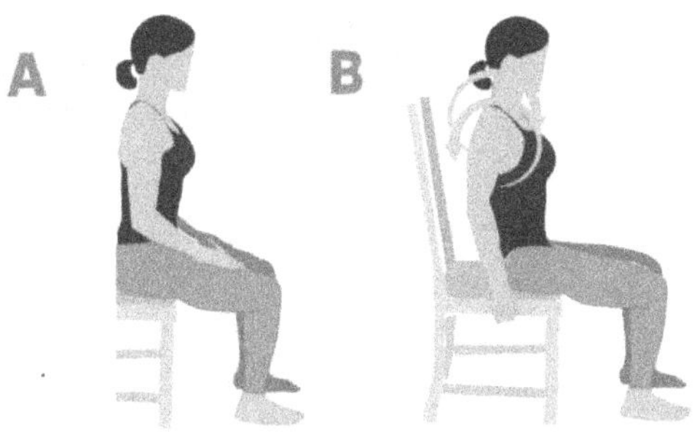

Shoulder rolls

Shoulder Rolls with Hands

1. Just like your regular shoulder roll, start in Mountain pose, but place your fingertips on your shoulders.

2. Make slow circles with your shoulders, using your elbows as your guide. You can go faster if

that feels good, but start slow and notice your breath as you complete each circle.

3. Do five complete circles in one direction, then reverse your circles and do five more.

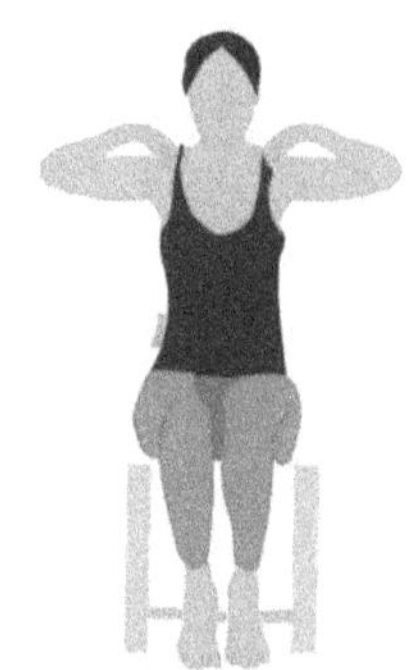

Shoulder rolls with hands

Seated Side Twist

1. Find your seated Mountain pose and maintain a nice straight back with your shoulders relaxed and away from your ears.

2. As you breathe in, gently twist to the right. Place your left hand on your right knee and let your right hand find any spot behind you that is comfortable. Turn your head to your right, bringing your gaze to rest gently over or toward your right shoulder.

3. Take another inhale in your twist and try to sit up straighter. As you exhale, return to Mountain pose.

4. Inhale again, and now twist to your left, resting your right hand on your right knee. Focus on your breathing as you sit up tall. Breathe out and return to Mountain pose.

5. Complete this twist five times on each side.

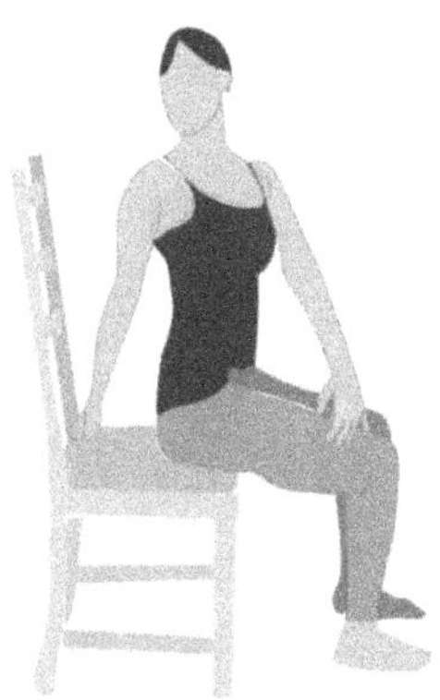

**Seated side
twist**

Volcano Arms

1. Come to sit in Mountain pose.

2. Inhale slowly and begin to lift both arms up and over your head in the shape of a V. Pay attention to your shoulders. If they are lifting up toward your ears, gently relax them down.

3. Breathe out and lower your arms back to your starting position.

4. Perform this pose at least three more times, matching your breathing to your movements. If you experience any discomfort as you lift your arms all the way up, only go as far as feels good without causing any pain.

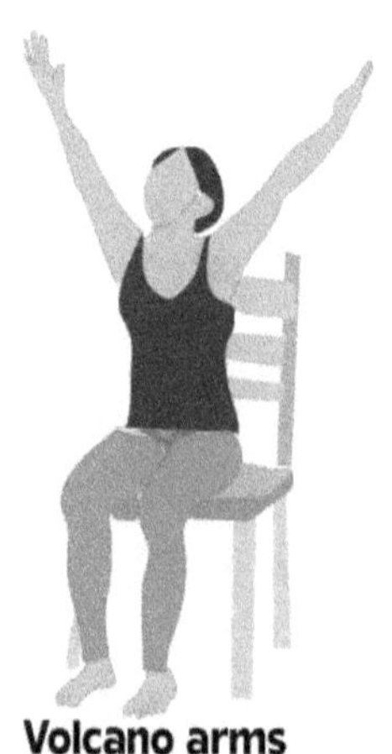

Volcano arms

Warrior II Arms

1. Begin in Mountain pose, sitting up tall with your feet firmly pressing into the floor. If you're slouching, you will diminish your breath, making the pose more difficult.

2. Extend both arms up and out to your sides until they are about shoulder level. Don't force your arms to go further than feels comfortable. If there is any discomfort or pain, lower your arms to a position where the feeling subsides.

3. Keeping your arms lifted, breathe in and squeeze your fingers into tight fists. On your exhale, open your fingers and stretch them as wide as you can, exaggerating the movement.

4. Lower your arms, returning to Mountain pose.

5. Do this movement about eight more times.

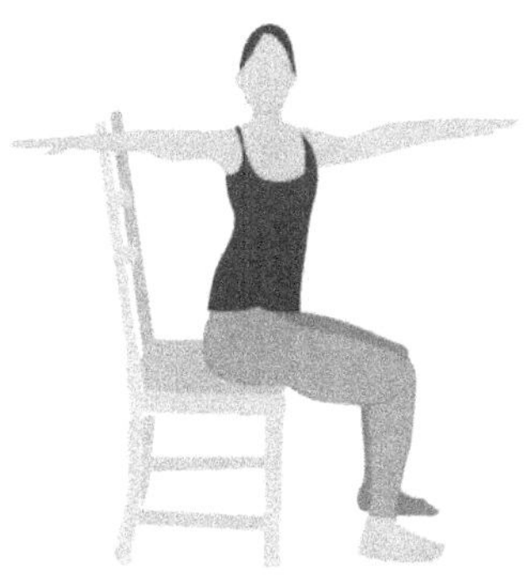

Warrior 2 arms

Eagle Arms

1. Start in Mountain pose with your knees hip-width apart and your feet pressing into the floor.

2. Inhale, and reach your arms up and out to your sides.

3. On an exhale, bring your arms forward in front of you, placing your right arm under your left arm and holding your shoulders with opposite hands, as if you're giving yourself a hug. If you have more mobility in your shoulders, you can continue wrapping your arms until the palms of your hands are touching each other, instead of your shoulders.

4. Breathe in and lift your arms a little higher. Exhale and release your arms back to your sides.

5. Repeat this movement on the other side with your left arm going under your right.

6. Practice this pose at least three times on each side.

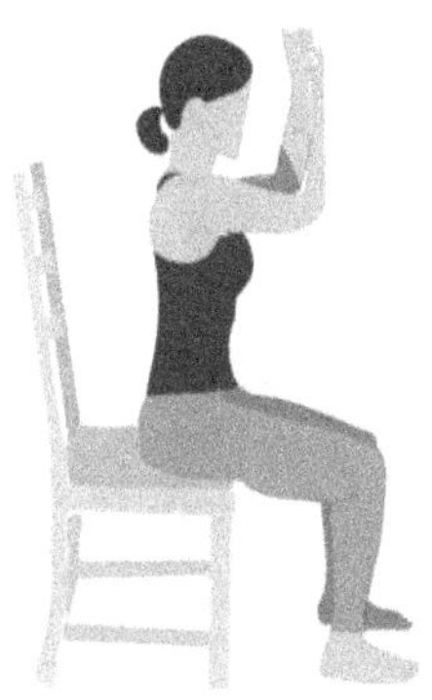

Eagle arms

Knee Swings

1. Come to Seated Mountain pose, with your belly button pulled in and your shoulders relaxed away from your ears.

2. If you can, interlace your fingers under your right knee for support and slowly begin to kick your right leg back and forth. If reaching under your knee is difficult, you can sit all the way back in your chair and kick your right leg back and forth.

3. Complete ten swings on your right side, then repeat these steps on your left side. As always, only lift your leg as high as feels comfortable and go at a pace that is sustainable for you. Also, make sure you check on your breathing.

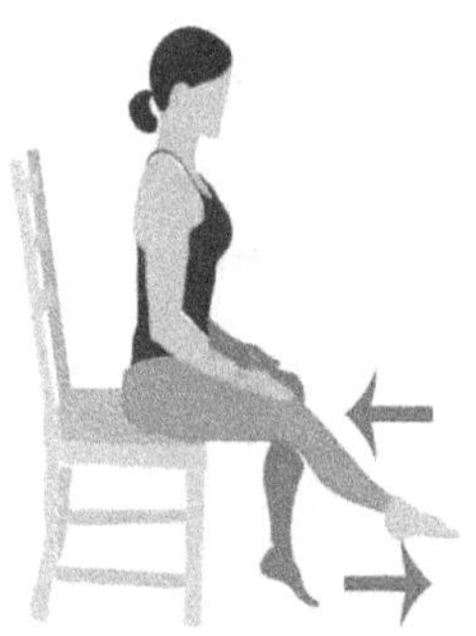

Knee swings

Leg Lifts With Point and Flex

1. Begin by sitting up tall in your chair with your feet firmly pressing into the ground. Place your hands anywhere that is comfortable.

2. On an inhale, extend your right leg out in front of you, keeping your left foot firmly on the floor. Only go as high or as far as feels good for you. With your leg extended off the floor, point and flex your right foot a few times. You can do this slowly or quickly, depending on how you feel.

3. On an exhale, slowly lower your right foot.

4. Do this at least five times on your right side, then switch and repeat on your left side. As you become stronger and more confident in your

movements, you can increase the number of lifts.

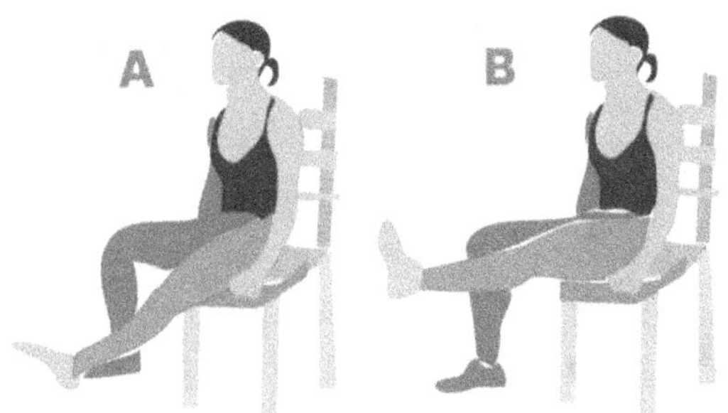

**Leg lifts with point
and flex**

Seated Forward Fold

1. Sit up tall in your chair with your feet flat on the floor and your toes pointing forward. Keep your knees hip-width apart and gently rest your palms on your thighs.

2. Keeping your back straight and your spine extended, inhale and begin to lean forward, hinging from your hips as if you're peering over a ledge. Go only as far as you can without rounding your back. You should feel a gentle stretch in your back and the backs of your legs.

3. Hold here for two breaths.

4. On your next exhale, using the muscles of your core and your hands for support, rise back up to a seated position.

5. Complete this motion at least five times. Your movements can be big or small and will depend on the flexibility of your spine and the mobility in your hips. As you strengthen and lengthen your muscles, you will increase your flexibility, as well as your mobility.

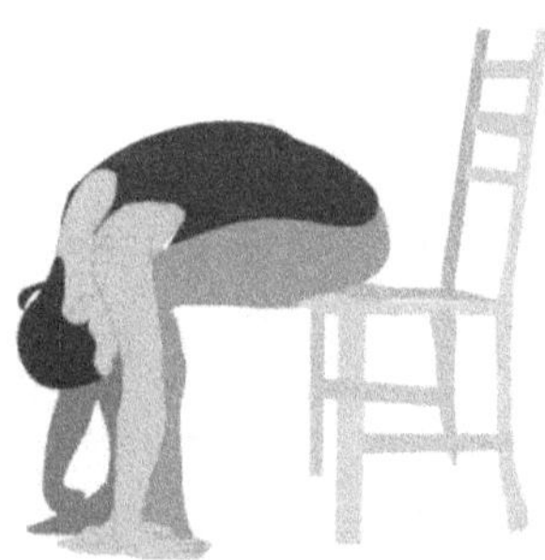

Seated forward fold

Seated Backbend

1. Sit in Mountain pose with your hands resting on the tops of your thighs, palms facing down.

2. Breathe in and slowly lift your chin up. Open your chest, pressing shoulder blades together, and slightly arch your back. You should be looking up toward the ceiling.

3. As you exhale, slowly lower your chin to your chest, dropping your head, and rounding your shoulders. You should be looking toward your belly button.

4. Repeat this movement five times, focusing on moving with your breath.

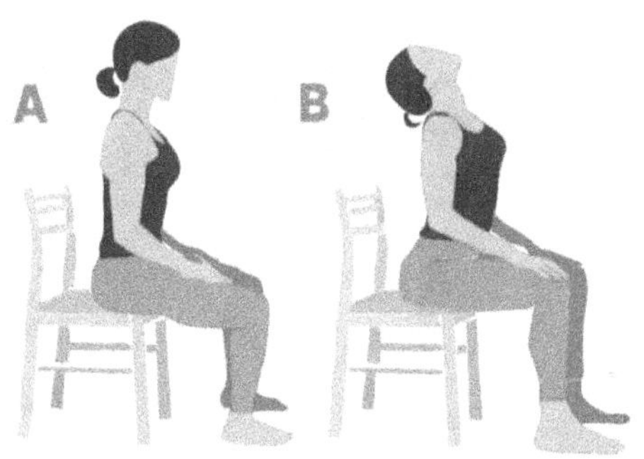

Seated backbend

Supported Chair Pose

1. Sit up tall in your chair with your knees hip-width apart and your feet flat on the floor, toes pointing forward. Place your hands on the sides of your chair.

2. Keeping your spine tall and your back straight, lean forward as if you're going into a seated forward fold. Try to keep your neck and spine in a straight line.

3. Leaning forward, slowly lift up out of your chair (about six inches) using your hands for support, then gently lower back down, returning to your seated position.

4. Perform this pose eight times.

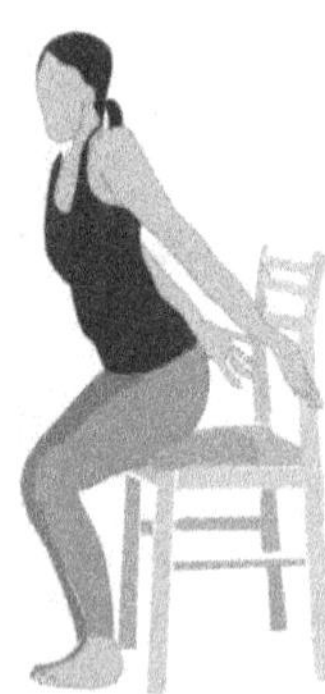

Supported chair pose

Full Body Stretch With Weights

1. Start in Mountain pose.

2. Hold a two-pound weight in each hand and rest your hands on your thighs, with your palms facing up.

3. As you inhale, lift your arms and legs up at the same time, keeping your back straight. If you feel like it is too difficult to stay sitting up

straight, lower your arms and legs a little until you feel like you can keep your back straight.

4. Hold here for one cycle of breath.

5. On an exhale, slowly lower your arms and legs back to your starting position.

6. Try to do this stretch at least eight times. Once you've completed the stretch, return to Mountain pose and observe your breath. Pay attention to how your body feels.

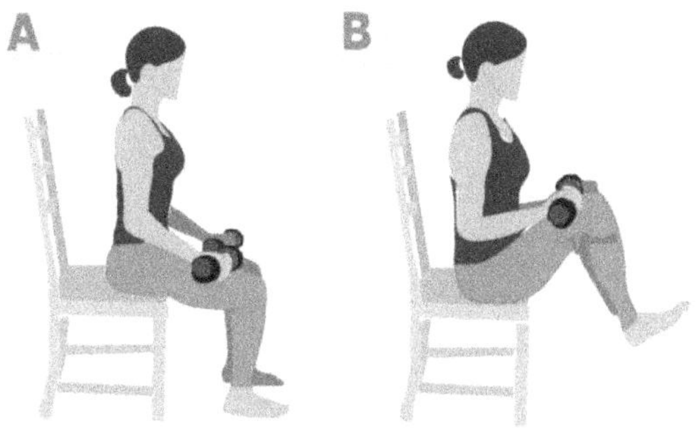

Full body stretch with weights

Conclusion

You've reached the end of the book, but hopefully it's just the beginning of your journey. I know that every day is different and each day your body feels differently. It is important to know that there may be days that you struggle to find the motivation to be active—and that's okay. You and your body need different things on different days. This is a process of experimentation and learning and discovering what works best for you. This book was created as a practical guide that is within your reach, and clearly outlines the steps you need to take in order to become a healthier, stronger version of yourself.

It is my sincere hope that by embracing the tips, tools, guidelines, and resources I have shared here, you are not only able to become stronger, but find the confidence in yourself and your ability to be happier and more independent. The goal here is to work on achieving mental, physical, and emotional wellness. Once you've gotten that, it will have a positive impact; not only on you, but also on those around you.

Throughout the book, we have provided different routines and modifications to those routines to assist you with working on finding that strength and challenging yourself to move more. We started by focusing on our mind, our emotions, and how we perceive ourselves because, as you know, in order to truly overcome our obstacles, we must focus on who we are in this moment, and determine what we need to do to move beyond those obstacles.

Though it may seem easier to avoid the harder, more challenging things, avoidance is not the solution. If your goal is to lead a more independent life that allows you to perform your daily tasks and do the things you enjoy most, then you need to use the tools provided here to realize them. In the end, you will feel a greater sense of accomplishment and take pride in your self-sufficiency.

Choose Your Path, Fulfill Your Goals

I know as you get older it seems like you are not only losing your independence, but also your choices. We have already established that age is just a number. You may not be able to change your chronological age, but you most certainly can determine your biological age. It is your responsibility to take charge of yourself and your needs, and do what's right for your life. Only you can decide how you are feeling, and only you can understand how your decisions affect your independence and mobility.

I challenge you to recognize your strength and determination as a person, as a senior, and as a contributing member of society. Once you've recognized your worth, value yourself and how much you still have to give and accomplish, regardless of your age. Make the time and the space to check in with yourself, and to nurture and nourish your mind, body, and spirit. Your strength and determination come from understanding and appreciating your worth. It is only by doing these things that you can begin to achieve your goals of strength, flexibility, mobility, and ultimately, independence.

Prioritize your physical fitness and ensure that it is a part of your daily routine. Eliminate those thoughts of self-doubt in your capabilities. They add no value and will keep you from achieving your end results. Motivate yourself and surround yourself with friends who have similar aims. This will help to build your confidence, and when you are more confident mentally, it can translate into confidence in your abilities, meaning you will be at less risk of injury when you complete your daily tasks or when you play with your grandkids. Finding the time now to develop your exercise routine means that you have many years ahead of you to spend with your loved ones, doing what you enjoy without the worry of being a burden.

We know that, as older adults, we worry constantly about being reliant on our loved ones for our day-to-day needs. Being physically strong and moving daily can help to ease some of that worry, but we also need to fortify ourselves mentally. Begin and end your day with a few moments of quiet. Take those moments to be with yourself and to assess how your body feels and how your mind feels. Our society has created many generalizations about what it means to age and to be older, but we know that there is a difference. Break that mold, and live your life freely and independently.

We should seize the opportunity to make our journey our own and to truly probe what getting older means to us, and for us. How do we find our own value as we age? What steps will you take to find your stronger, more independent self?

What Happens Next?

You've taken the first step by reading this book all the way to the end. You understand better now how aging works, and which parts of the process you can and cannot control. The question is, now: Are you willing and ready to control the things that you can? Do you want to get up easily from your seat, play with your grandkids, do your own groceries, and generally live your own life without pain and without the fear of falling or injury?

If your answer is yes to any or all of these questions, then I'm fairly certain you know what you need to do next. First off, be sure to book an appointment with your doctor. As you know, any changes to your physical routine should be discussed with a healthcare professional to ensure that you are doing what's safe for you. Once you've gotten the green light medically, then I highly recommend you take the time to go through the ritual of preparing your space and getting your gear. It may seem like a small thing, but doing this makes you invested in the outcomes, and in some ways, can get you excited about starting your routine.

Try to enlist some friends or family members. Exercising is always more fun when you have company. Once you're all set, choose a time and a routine that suits you and your fitness level. As you get stronger, you can always add on more. Make sure to warm up and cool down and add some music to create ambience. Stay hydrated and pay attention to how your body feels. Don't overdo it; it's not worth being injured. Whatever physical activity or routine you choose, be sure that you commit to it. It won't work if you just do it once in a while. Most importantly, have fun! So, what are you waiting for... ?

References

American Seniors Community. (2015, December 8). *The best core exercises for seniors.* Senior Living Communities & Nursing Homes in Indiana | ASC. https://www.asccare.com/the-best-core-exercises-for-seniors/

Balbim, G. (n.d.). *Physical activity for older adults: It's never too late to improve your health.* Society of Behavioral Medicine. Retrieved July 2, 2022, from https://www.sbm.org/healthy-living/physical-activity-for-older-adults-its-never-too-late-to-improve-your-health?gclid=CjwKCAjw682TBhATEiwA9crl3 74gThHTZXU06VIZyKZX1a31SiMbJ4OiCtE RY3P5Wtg4kQfNJFBerhoC18kQAvD_BwE

Basaraba, S. (2021, November 10). *How smoking causes early aging and premature wrinkles.* Verywell Mind. https://www.verywellmind.com/how-smoking-ages-skin-2223424#:~:text=to%20quit%20smoking.-

Benedictine. (2021, September 15). *5 easy and fun ways to stay active as you age.* Benedictine. https://www.benedictineliving.org/blog/5-easy-and-fun-ways-to-stay-active-as-you-age/?utm_term=how%20to%20stay%20healthy &utm_caresources

Campbell, B. J. (2020). *Exercise and bone health.* Aaos.org. https://orthoinfo.aaos.org/en/staying-healthy/exercise-and-bone-health/

Care As One. (2021a, April 12). *10 best knee strengthening exercises for seniors.* Careasone Blog. https://careasone.com/blog/10-best-knee-strengthening-exercises-for-seniors/

Care As One. (2021b, June 16). *10 best back strengthening exercises for seniors.* Careasone Blog. https://careasone.com/blog/10-best-back-strengthening-exercises-for-seniors/

CDC. (2019). *Keep on your feet.* Centers for Disease Control and Prevention. https://www.cdc.gov/injury/features/older-adult-falls/index.html

The Center Foundation. (2020, October 13). *Warm up for injury prevention and performance.* The Center Foundation. https://www.centerfoundation.org/warm-up-for-injury-prevention/?gclid=Cj0KCQjwpcOTBhCZARIsAEAYLuUMLfrCjeN_o7FADEzk2wiiH9Centers for Disease Control. (2021a, May 5). Older adults. Www.cdc.gov.

https://www.cdc.gov/stillgoingstrong/olderadu
lts/index.html

Centers for Disease Control. (2021b, June 4). *Still going
strong campaign.* Www.cdc.gov.
https://www.cdc.gov/stillgoingstrong/index.ht
ml

Centers for Disease Control and Prevention. (2019).
How much physical activity do older adults need?
Cdc.gov.
https://www.cdc.gov/physicalactivity/basics/o
lder_adults/index.htm

Centers for Disease Control and Prevention. (2020,
November 23). *Knowing is not enough—act on your
family health history.* Www.cdc.gov.
https://www.cdc.gov/genomics/famhistory/kn
owing_not_enough.htm

Cherry, K. (2013, August 14). *Adult neurogenesis and the
science of new brain cell regeneration.* Verywell Mind;
Verywell Mind.
https://www.verywellmind.com/adult-
neurogenesis-can-we-grow-new-brain-cells-
2794885

Cleveland Clinic. (2021, August 17). *Why senior mobility is
so important right now.* Cleveland Clinic.
https://health.clevelandclinic.org/why-senior-
mobility-is-so-important-right-now/

Coach Sofia Fitness. (2020, June 30). *8 standing core exercises for back pain.* Coach Sofia Fitness. https://www.coachsofiafitness.com/8-standing-core-exercises-for-back-pain/

Cruz Lemar, M. (2019, October 29). *Here's why it is never too late to get yourself active.* The Independent. https://www.independent.co.uk/news/science/exercise-keeping-active-health-benefits-heart-elderly-a9171016.html

DeSimone, N. (2021, May 14). *Alcohol and aging effects: Does alcohol make you look older?* Kingsway Recovery. https://kingswayrecovery.com/alcohol-and-aging-effects/#:~:text=Dehydration%20can%20sap%20your%20skin

DuVall, J. (2016, August 18). *3 breathing techniques for a more effective workout.* Life by Daily Burn. https://dailyburn.com/life/fitness/breathing-techniques-strength-training/

Exercises For Injuries. (2016, May 27). *4 best lower back pain stretching exercises while standing.* Www.youtube.com. https://www.youtube.com/watch?v=Bu4EuPsrdvQ&ab_channel=ExercisesForInjuries

Ferreira, M. (2017, July 27). *Why you need music when you exercise.* Healthline.

https://www.healthline.com/health/music-can-make-or-break-your-workout#Bottom-line-

Fetters, K. A., & Esposito, L. (2020, September 30). *12 best equipment-free exercises for older adults.* US News. https://health.usnews.com/health-news/health-wellness/articles/best-equipment-free-strength-exercises-for-older-adults

Gregory, N. (2021, July 9). *Brain exercises that work.* Forbes Health. https://www.forbes.com/health/healthy-aging/brain-exercises/

Harrison, E. (2022, February 22). *Aging lungs: Breathing exercises you can do at home to increase lung capacity.* SeniorsMatter. https://www.seniorsmatter.com/aging-lungs-breathing-exercises-you-can-do-at-home/2597844/

Harvard Health Publishing. (2021, April 1). *The best core exercises for older adults.* Harvard Health. https://www.health.harvard.edu/staying-healthy/the-best-core-exercises-for-older-adults

Healthline. (n.d.). *How to strengthen wrists: Stretches, exercises, and tips.* Healthline. https://www.healthline.com/health/how-to-strengthen-wrists

Healthline. (2014, August 14). *5 seated back pain stretches for seniors.* Healthline. https://www.healthline.com/health/back-pain/stretches-for-seniors

Healthline. (2018, September 17). *You can do this low-impact cardio workout in 20 minutes.* Healthline. https://www.healthline.com/health/fitness-exercise/low-impact-cardio

Healthline. (2020, March 10). *Seated and standing chair exercises for seniors.* Healthline. https://www.healthline.com/health/chair-exercises-for-seniors

Healthline. (2021, March 23). *Why do we age, and can anything be done to stop or slow it?* Healthline. https://www.healthline.com/health/why-do-we-age

Healthy Human. (n.d.). *Science-backed reasons why exercise makes you younger.* Healthy Human. https://healthyhumanlife.com/blogs/news/exercise-makes-you-younger

Higley, S. (2020b, August 25). *What effect does music have on exercise and your brain?* Campusrecreation.wvu.edu. https://campusrecreation.wvu.edu/news/health-and-wellbeing/2020/08/25/what-effect-does-music-have-on-exercise-and-your-brain#:~:text=

Integrated Rehabilitation Services. (2021, April 15). *Benefits of increasing upper body strength.* Integrated Rehabilitation Services. https://integrehab.com/blog/strength-and-conditioning/upper-body-strength/

Iora With One Medical. (2020, October 8). *Yoga for seniors: 5 easy poses you can do at home.* Iora Primary Care. https://ioraprimarycare.com/blog/yoga-for-seniors-poses-at-home/

Iora With One Medical. (2021, January 21). *9 hip strengthening exercises for seniors.* Iora Primary Care. https://ioraprimarycare.com/blog/hip-strengthening-exercises-for-seniors/

ISSA. (2020, June 18). *Top six exercises for building bigger calves.* Www.issaonline.com. https://www.issaonline.com/blog/post/top-six-exercises-for-building-bigger-calves

Kovar, E. (2015, December 7). *Music and exercise: How music affects exercise motivation.* Www.acefitness.org. https://www.acefitness.org/resources/everyone/blog/5763/music-and-exercise-how-music-affects-exercise-motivation/

Levine, D. (n.d.). *Foot and ankle exercises for seniors.* Davidslevinemd.com. Retrieved July 2, 2022, from https://davidslevinemd.com/foot-and-ankle-exercises-for-seniors

Mayo Clinic. (2020, August 11). *Slide show: Exercises to improve your core strength.* Mayo Clinic. https://www.mayoclinic.org/healthy-lifestyle/fitness/multimedia/core-strength/sls-20076575?s=13

McCoy, J. (2018, September 22). *Here's why the way you breathe during a workout matters.* SELF. https://www.self.com/story/how-to-breathe-during-a-workout

Med Mart. (2021, June 21). *5 lower body exercises lying down - senior exercises at home.* Www.youtube.com. https://www.youtube.com/watch?v=gCGbL8bs-Go&ab_channel=MedMart

MedLine Plus. (2021, May 12). *Why is it important to know my family medical history?* Medlineplus.gov. https://medlineplus.gov/genetics/understanding/inheritance/familyhistory/

More Life Health. (n.d.). *Great lower body exercise library for seniors.* More Life Health - Seniors Health & Fitness. https://morelifehealth.com/ll-exercise-library

More Life Health Seniors. (2018, October 3). *Seated lower back exercises for seniors.* Www.youtube.com. https://www.youtube.com/watch?v=XTEfL12pli8&ab_channel=MoreLifeHealthSeniors

More Life Health Seniors. (2019, March 31). *Standing warm-up routine for seniors (do before undertaking exercise)*. Www.youtube.com. https://www.youtube.com/watch?v=b2DYU7 ZQgN0&ab_channel=MoreLifeHealthSeniors

National Institute on Aging. (2017). *Facts about aging and alcohol*. National Institute on Aging. https://www.nia.nih.gov/health/facts-about-aging-and-alcohol

Pain Relief Institute. (2019, March 20). *Shoulder exercises for seniors*. Pain Relief Institute. https://www.painfreepainrelief.com/shoulder-exercises-for-seniors/#:~:text=To%20begin%2C%20stand%20or%20sit

Shrift, D. (n.d.). *Elbow exercises for seniors and the elderly*. Eldergym. https://eldergym.com/elbow-exercises/

Silver Sneakers. (2020, March 21). *Tone your trouble spots: Thighs*. SilverSneakers. https://www.silversneakers.com/blog/thigh-exercises-older-adults/#:~:text=Thigh%20Exercise%20%231%3A%20Sit-to-Stand&text=From%2

Silver Sneakers. (2022, April 26). *Neck stretches for seniors: 4 ways to prevent neck pain*. SilverSneakers. https://www.silversneakers.com/blog/4-neck-

stretches-you-should-do-right-now-even-if-
your-neck-feels-fine/

Stannah UK. (2017, April 5). *6 basic wrist exercises for
seniors.* Www.youtube.com.
https://www.youtube.com/watch?v=v0XI_5J9
5EU&ab_channel=StannahUK

Sunny Health and Fitness. (202 C.E., April 15). *Upper
body exercise benefits.* Sunny Health and Fitness.
https://sunnyhealthfitness.com/blogs/health-
wellness/upper-body-exercise-benefits

Sunshine Retirement Living. (2016, December 19). *7
remarkable reasons to encourage & promote senior
mobility.* Sunshine Retirement Living.
https://www.sunshineretirementliving.com/hea
lth-wellness/7-remarkable-reasons-encourage-
promote-senior-
mobility/#:~:text=According%20to%20the%2
0CDC%2C%20regular

Sweat. (2019, October 31). *Low-intensity cardio training:
What is it & how does it work?* SWEAT.
https://www.sweat.com/blogs/fitness/low-
intensity-cardio

Web MD. (n.d.). *Benefits of annual checkups in your 50's and
older.* WebMD.
https://www.webmd.com/healthy-
aging/annual-checkups-seniors-importance#1

Webb, L. M., & Chen, C. Y. (2021). *The COVID19 pandemic's impact on older adults' mental health: Contributing factors, coping strategies, and opportunities for improvement.* International Journal of Geriatric Psychiatry, 37(1). https://doi.org/10.1002/gps.5647

Yoga With Adriene. (2018, June 3). *Yoga for seniors | Slow and gentle yoga.* Www.youtube.com. https://www.youtube.com/watch?v=kFhG-ZzLNN4&ab_channel=YogaWithAdriene